Coagulation
Problems during
Pregnancy

CURRENT REVIEW IN OBSTETRICS AND GYNAECOLOGY

OBSTETRICS

Series Editor
Tom Lind MB BS DSc PhD MRCPath MRCOG
MRC Human Reproduction Group, Princess Mary Maternity Hospital, Newcastle upon Tyne

Volumes published
Obstetric Analgesia and Anaesthesia *J. Selwyn Crawford*
Early Diagnosis of Fetal Defects *D. J. J. Brock*
Early Teenage Pregnancy *J. K. Russell*
Aspects of Care in Labour *J. M. Beazley and M. O. Lobb*
Drug Prescribing in Pregnancy *B. Krauer, F. Krauer and F. Hytten*
Spontaneous Abortion *H. J. Huisjes*

Volumes in preparation
Immunology of Pregnancy *W. Page Faulk and H. Fox*
Hypertension and Related Problems in Pregnancy *W. A. W. Walters*
Ultrasound in Obstetrics *W. J. Garrett and P. S. Warren*
Fetoscopy *C. H. Rodeck*
Diabetic Pregnancy *M. Brudenell and M. Dodderidge*

GYNAECOLOGY

Series Editors
Albert Singer DPhil PhD FRCOG
Whittington Hospital, London

Joe A. Jordan MD DObst FRCOG
Birmingham Maternity Hospital, Queen Elizabeth Medical Centre, Birmingham

Volumes published
Ovarian Malignancies *M. S. Piver*
Cancer of the Cervix *H. M. Shingleton and J. Orr*
Female Puberty and its Abnormalities *J. Dewhurst*

Volumes in preparation
Therapeutic Abortion *A. A. Calder*
Male Infertility *A. M. Jequier*
Gynaecological Premalignant Disease *A. Singer, F. Sharp and J. Jordon*
The Menopause *M. Thom*
Urinary Incontinence *S. L. R. Stanton, L. Cardozo and P. Hilton*
Endometriosis *D. O'Connor*
Endocrine Aspects of Female Infertility *M. Hull*

Elizabeth A. Letsky

MB BS FRCPath

Consultant Haematologist, Queen Charlotte's
Hospital for Women, and Hospital for Sick Children,
Great Ormond Street, London

Coagulation Problems during Pregnancy

Series Editor

TOM LIND

CHURCHILL LIVINGSTONE

EDINBURGH LONDON MELBOURNE AND NEW YORK 1985

CHURCHILL LIVINGSTONE
Medical Division of Longman Group Limited

Distributed in the United States of America by Churchill
Livingstone Inc., 1560 Broadway, New York, N.Y. 10036,
and by associated companies, branches and representatives
throughout the world.

First published 1985
Reprinted 1985

ISBN 0 443 02360 3
ISSN 0264-5610

British Library Cataloguing in Publication Data

Letsky, Elizabeth A.
    Coagulation problems during pregnancy.——
    (Current reviews in obstetrics and gynecology,
    ISSN 0264-5610)
    1. Pregnancy, Complications of   2. Blood——
    Coagulation, Disorders of
    I. Title   II. Series
    618.3'261   RG580.B5

Library of Congress Cataloging in Publication Data

Letsky, Elizabeth A.
    Coagulation problems during pregnancy.

    (Current reviews in obstetrics and gynaecology)
    Includes bibliographies and index.
    1. Blood—Coagulation, Disorders of.   2. Pregnancy,
Complications of.   I. Title.   II. Series.   [DNLM:
1. Blood Coagulation Disorders—in pregnancy.
W1 CU8093M / WH 322 L649c]
RG580.B56L48   1984   618.3   84-12053

Printed in Great Britain by
Butler & Tanner Ltd, Frome and London

Foreword

Some years ago when visiting obstetric units in another country I was surprised to find the young obstetricians requesting a 'clotting screen' on virtually every woman admitted to the antenatal or labour wards with a vaginal bleed no matter how small or symptomless. This was not the routine practice in the UK at the time and prompted me to ask what the expected incidence of true clotting disorders was likely to be in an average antenatal population and what proportion of women with antepartum bleeding would be likely to have such a haematological condition as the cause. Several subsidiary questions arose: which tests are included in such 'clotting screens'; how effective are they for pregnant women; do any commonly taken drugs affect such tests; how cost-effective are they; and do they actually influence management. I did not know the answers and my only comfort was that my ignorance seemed to be shared by the doctors requesting the tests! When Churchill Livingstone asked me to edit the series this topic seemed an essential choice because I find that while the practice of requesting these blood tests has now spread to the UK the true understanding of their meaning and influence upon patient management seems to have been left behind.

Dr Letsky is not only an experienced haematologist but has taken a specific interest in the haematological problems associated with pregnancy and young children. She has the added advantage of having used part of her early career to train in obstetrics and gynaecology and as this training was in Newcastle the foundations must have been soundly laid! When inviting her to write this book I asked that the needs of the obstetrician be borne in mind with emphasis on such details as which tests were appropriate to a given circumstance and even the types of sample tubes which should be used. As with any specialist subject it is not easy for those already skilled in its practice to write for those requiring rather basic information but Dr Letsky has done the job admirably. I am sure the book will be a valuable addition to the bookshelves of all who care for pregnant women.

Newcastle upon Tyne   Tom Lind
1985

Preface

Haemorrhage and thrombosis are major hazards for the pregnant woman. There are few texts available which span the whole field from the unique physiology of haemostasis in normal pregnancy, to the wide spectrum of clinical problems which may occur, the interactions of acquired and genetic disorders, their clinical and laboratory investigation and management.

An attempt to provide a book of manageable and useful size for those involved in the clinical diagnosis and management of obstetric patients with haemostatic problems has been made. It is hoped that it will provide information and guidance to all those interested in this field and while not being fully comprehensive, will at least point them in the right direction to gain more knowledge of conditions of specific interest.

If I were to express gratitude to everyone who has helped me during the lengthy gestation of this rather brief tome, the acknowledgments would be longer than the text, but I must pick out one or two individuals for special thanks for the particularly valuable assistance they have given me.

First, my small but loyal staff at Queen Charlotte's Maternity Hospital, who have put up with my pre-occupation and irritability with stoicism and cheerfulness over the past few months.

Numerous clinical colleagues have given me the benefit of their expertise and educated me in the many areas where my knowledge is lacking. Of these, Dr Mica Brozovic has always been prepared to lend a critical ear and give constructive advice. Professor Murdo Elder, Dr Reuben Mibashan and Professor E. R. Huehns pointed me in the way of valuable references and Dr Michael de Swiet is largely responsible for much of the content of the chapter on thromboembolism.

Professor R. M. Hardisty has taken some of his valuable time to check that there are no clottish gaffes in the text.

As far as preparing the manuscript is concerned I am totally indebted to my clairvoyant secretary, Audrey Tapley, who was able to decipher my incredibly bizarre handwriting and was unfailingly good humoured throughout my frequent grumpy periods, and to John Arthur who painstakingly prepared the figures and has always been ready with constructive suggestions.

Most of all I feel I must express my gratitude to my mother whose timely severe illness from which she has mercifully completely recovered, delayed the completion of the text so that important 1983 references could be included.

London
1985

Elizabeth A. Letsky

Contents

Haemostasis and tests of the integrity of haemostatic systems in health

Haemostasis in health

Introduction

This necessarily brief section is not a comprehensive account of normal haemostasis and tests of haemostatic function, but is intended to give those involved in obstetric practice a reasonable basis on which to build an understanding of haemostatic competence, its investigation and the physiological changes in the systems involved in coagulation and fibrinolysis, which occur during pregnancy.

For convenience many of the references given pertain to obstetric practice and are not necessarily key scientific references of pioneer work in the field. For a practical clinical text of manageable size which deals with current theories of healthy haemostasis and the investigation of haemostatic failure in more detail the reader is referred to a publication of Ingram & colleagues (1982). Those who require even more information about haemostasis in health and disease, including a relatively small chapter concerning haemostatic disorders during pregnancy (Bonnar 1981), will find all they need contained in a large tome entitled *Haemostasis and Thrombosis* (Bloom & Thomas 1981).

Haemostasis and Fibrinolysis

The integrity and patency of the vascular tree is dependent upon finely controlled interactions between the platelets and the vessel wall and between the coagulation system and fibrinolysis. During pregnancy major changes occur in the components of the haemostatic system, and some of the physiological adaptations are

1

unique to human pregnancy. However, their significance and relationship to haemorrhage and thrombosis — both major hazards for the pregnant woman — can only be appreciated with a knowledge of the haemostatic mechanism in the healthy nonpregnant individual.

Haemostasis

Haemostasis in health has three primary functions:
  1. To confine the circulating blood to the vascular bed.
  2. To maintain its fluidity.
  3. To arrest bleeding from injured vessels.
All these aspects of haemostasis depend on a complex interaction between vasculature, platelets, coagulation factors and fibrinolysis.

Vascular integrity, platelets and prostacyclin

It is not known how vascular integrity is normally maintained, but it is clear that the platelets have a key role to play because conditions in which their number is depleted or their function is abnormal are characterised by widespread spontaneous capillary haemorrhages. It is thought that in health the platelets constantly are sealing microdefects of the vasculature, minifibrin clots being formed and then unwanted fibrin being removed by a process of fibrinolysis.

Prostaglandins are vaso-active substances with a wide variety of other actions in mammalian species. The main precursor of prostaglandins in man is the polyunsaturated fatty acid arachidonic acid (Fig. 1.1). For many years it was thought that the only products of arachidonic acid metabolism were chemically stable prosta-glandins such as PGE_2 and $PGF_{2\alpha}$. In recent years unstable derivatives of arachidonic acid have been found to be of importance especially with relation to maintenance of vascular integrity involving platelets and the vessel wall (Moncada & Vane 1981). In platelets, arachidonic acid is mainly converted into an unstable vasoconstrictor and platelet aggregating substance — thromboxane A_2 (TXA_2).

Prostacyclin (PGI_2) is an unstable prostaglandin first described by Moncada & colleagues in 1976. It is the principal prostanoid synthesised by blood vessels and is a powerful vasodilator and potent inhibitor of platelet aggregation. Moncada & Vane (1979) have proposed that there is a balance between the production of prostacyclin by the vessel walls and the production of the

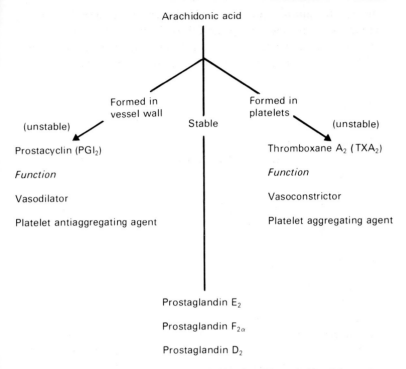

Fig. 1.1 The prostaglandins derived from arachidonic acid metabolism (after Moncada & Vane 1979).

vasoconstrictor and powerful aggregating agent thromboxane by the platelets. Prostacyclin prevents aggregation at much lower concentrations than is needed to prevent adhesion and therefore vascular damage leads to platelet adhesion but not necessarily to aggregation and subsequent thrombus formation.

When the injury is minor small platelet thrombi form and are washed away by the circulation as described above, but the extent of the injury is an important determinant of the size of the thrombus and whether or not platelet aggregation is stimulated. Prostacyclin synthetase is abundant in the intima of the vessel walls and progressively decreases in concentration from the intima to the adventitia. In contrast the proaggregating elements increase in concentration from the subendothelium to the adventitia. It follows that severe vessel damage will lead to the development of a large thrombus as opposed to simple platelet adherence.

Aspirin and other similar drugs have been known to inhibit

thromboxane production by the platelet for many years (Vane 1971) and aspirin has been widely promoted as an antithrombotic drug. It has now become clear that aspirin and aspirin-like drugs can also inhibit the formation of prostacyclin by the vessel wall; the effect achieved appears to be dose dependent, very small doses having the desired effect of selectively suppressing production of thromboxane by the platelet.

It has been suggested (Moncada & Vane 1978) that drugs which can selectively inhibit TXA_2 formation will be superior to aspirin in the prevention and treatment of thrombo-embolism. Several such inhibitors have been found and are undergoing active investigation (Moncada & Vane 1981).

Deficiency of prostacyclin production has been observed in certain platelet consumption syndromes such as haemolytic uraemic syndrome and thrombotic thrombocytopenic purpura (Remuzzi et al 1978) and may play a part in their pathogenesis (see Ch. 5).

Arrest of bleeding

An essential requirement of the haemostatic system is a rapid reaction to injury, the effect of which remains confined to the area of damage. This requires control mechanisms which stimulate coagulation after trauma but limit the extent of the response. The substances involved in the formation of the haemostatic plug normally circulate in the blood in an inert form until activated at the site of vascular injury or by some factor released into the circulation which triggers off intravascular coagulation.

When a small blood vessel is injured the first recognisable event is the adherence of the platelets to the collagen in the exposed subendothelium of the vessel wall. This adherence triggers off a series of alterations in the platelets which can be shown in vitro and include formation of pseudopodia, change of shape and the release of constituents such as adenosine diphosphate (ADP) serotonin, calcium and secreted platelet proteins (Niewarowski 1981). Many of the substances released are of obvious haemostatic importance and include thromboxane, β thromboglobulin, fibrinogen, factor V and factor VIII related antigen, but platelets can also modify the functions of other cells, particularly the endothelial cells of the vessel wall by releasing a number of platelet proteins e.g. growth factors and vascular permeability factor. In this way platelets play a vital role in a number of processes influencing replication of endothelial cells, tissue repair, wound healing and inflammation. (Hardisty 1982).

ADP release increases the platelet plug by stimulating further aggregation of the platelets at the site of injury. Serotonin release promotes vasoconstriction and also stimulates further aggregation. The coagulation cascade is triggered off and the action of thrombin leads to the formation of fibrin which in turn converts the loose platelet plug into a firm stable wound seal. In the repair of small endothelial breaks in the microvasculature, platelets alone are probably enough to prevent haemorrhage. The role of platelets is of less importance in injury involving large vessels because platelet aggregates are of insufficient size and strength to breach the defect. Here the coagulation mechanism is of major importance in conjunction with vascular constriction.

The platelet contractile protein ('thrombosthenin') which is similar to muscle actomyosin is required not only for the secretion of active principles from the platelet (see above) but for the subsequent clot retraction. This helps to bring together injured edges and to clear the vascular lumen and allow blood flow to continue.

Blood coagulation

The end result of blood coagulation is the formation of an insoluble fibrin clot from the soluble precursor fibrinogen in the plasma. This involves a complex interaction of clotting factors and a sequential activation of a series of proenzymes. The original enzyme cascade of the coagulation system proposed by Macfarlane (1964) has been modified as a result of the recognition of complexes which form between certain activated factors.

A list of the clotting factors using their assigned Roman numeral and some of their alternative names is given in Table 1.1.

When a blood vessel is injured, blood coagulation is initiated by activation of factor XII by collagen (intrinsic mechanism) and activation of factor VII by thromboplastin release (extrinsic mechanism) from the damaged tissue. Both the intrinsic and extrinsic mechanisms are activated by components of the vessel wall and both are required for normal haemostasis. The two mechanisms are diagrammatically represented in Figure 1.2. Strict division between the two pathways does not exist and interactions between activated factors in both systems have been shown (Bonnar 1975). The combined pathways have been described as a biochemical amplifier. Coagulation factors present in picogram amounts stimulate a sequential series of enzyme conversions leading to the conversion of milligrams of fibrinogen to fibrin. The intrinsic and extrinsic systems

5

Coagulation Problems During Pregnancy

Table 1.1 Nomenclature of clotting factors

Factor	Synonyms
I	Fibrinogen
II	Prothrombin
[III]	Thromboplastin (tissue extract)
[IV]	Calcium
V	[Proaccelerin, labile factor, plasma ac-globulin]
[VI]	[Accelerin, a hypothetical intermediate product of the coagulation process]
VII	[Proconvertin, stable factor, serum prothrombin conversion accelerator (SPCA), cothromboplastin, autoprothrombin I]
VIII	Antihaemophilic factor (AHF), antihaemophilic globulin (AHG), antihaemophilic factor A
VIII:C	The coagulant activity of factor VIII as measured by clotting tests
VIII:CAg	The antigen detected by alloantibody (antibody arising in a treated haemophiliac)
VIIIR:Ag	The VIII-related antigen detected by xenoantibody (e.g. rabbit): VIII-related protein
IX	Christmas factor, antihaemophilic factor B, [plasma thromboplastin component (PTC) plasma thromboplastin factor B, beta-prothromboplastin, platelet cofactor 2, autoprothrombin II]
X	[Stuart-prower factor]
XI	Plasma thromboplastin antecedent (PTA) [antihaemophilic factor C, plasma thromboplastin factor C]
XII	Hageman factor
XIII	Fibrin stabilising factor (FSF)

[] Numbers or names now seldom used
After Ingram et al (1982)

share a common pathway, following the activation of factor X. The intrinsic pathway, or contact system, proceeds spontaneously and is relatively slow, requiring from 5 to 20 minutes for visible fibrin formation (Bonnar 1978). All tissues contain a specific lipoprotein, thromboplastin, which markedly increases the rate at which blood clots, but it is particularly concentrated in the lung and brain. The placenta also is very rich in tissue factor and small amounts of placenta added to the blood will produce fibrin formation within 12 seconds. This acceleration of coagulation by the tissue factor system is brought about by bypassing all the reactions involving the contact system.

The final steps in the clotting reactions for both systems involve the conversion of prothrombin to thrombin and the action of thrombin on fibrinogen. Fibrinogen is the only clotting factor present in

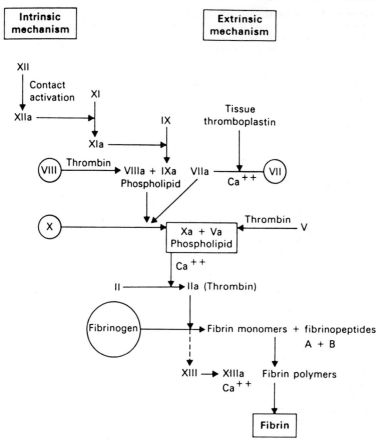

Fig. 1.2 The factors involved in blood coagulation and their interactions. The circled factors show significant increases in pregnancy.

sufficient quantity to allow its measurement in terms of milligrams of protein. Plasma levels in health lie between 2.5 and 4.0 g of fibrinogen per litre. The molecular weight of fibrinogen is approximately 344 000 and the molecule consists of three pairs of polypeptide chains linked by means of disulphide bonds. Thrombin, a proteolytic enzyme, splits off two pairs of small peptides (fibrinopeptide A and B) to produce fibrin monomer (Fig. 1.2) The removal of fibrinopeptides A and B, which carry negative charges, allows polymerisation of fibrin monomer. Polymeric fibrin, unlike fibrin monomer, is insoluble and on electron microscopy appears as fibrin strands which have characteristic cross-striations. The fibrin polymer

7

is strengthened by the action of factor XIII (fibrin stabilising factor) which, by linking amino acids of adjacent areas of the polymerised fibrin, confers tensile strength and insolubility to the fibrin and provides a medium suitable for tissue repair. Bleeding after separation of the umbilical cord, delayed bleeding after trauma, defective healing of wounds and the formation of wide scars are characteristic of hereditary deficiency of factor XIII.

Natural inhibitors of coagulation

Blood coagulation is strictly confined to the site of tissue injury in normal circumstances. Powerful mechanisms must control progressive coagulation or dissemination beyond the site of trauma would lead to widespread vascular occlusion. The action of thrombin in vivo is controlled by a number of mechanisms particularly its absorption onto the locally formed fibrin and the presence in the plasma of a potent inhibitor, antithrombin III, an $\alpha 2$ globulin which destroys thrombin activity. This is a protein which potentiates the antithrombin action of heparin, sometimes known as heparin cofactor.

Natural inhibitors of the coagulant enzymes which are produced in the early phases of coagulation have also been described. An agent which inhibits activated factor X — anti Xa — has also been identified. Heparin potentiates the action of anti Xa, which may be identical to the $\alpha 2$ globulin, antithrombin III (Biggs et al 1970). This is the rationale for the use of low-dose heparin for prophylaxis in patients at risk of thrombo-embolic phenomena (see Ch.2), particularly postoperative thrombosis (Bonnar 1976).

Fibrinolysis

It has been proposed that coagulation and fibrinolysis exist in normal human plasma in a balanced state but there is still no generally agreed role for this system in the day to day maintenance of haemostasis (Gaffney 1981). The fibrinolytic enzyme system has four basic components — plasminogen, plasmin, activators and inhibitors (Fig. 1.3).

Fibrin and fibrinogen are digested by plasmin, a proteolytic enzyme derived from an inactive plasma precursor — plasminogen. Plasminogen is a β globin of molecular weight 90 000. Synthesis,

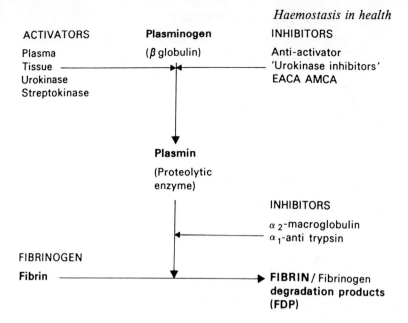

Fig. 1.3 Components of fibrinolytic system

most probably in the liver, can take place fairly rapidly, and treatment with streptokinase results in an increase in the plasminogen from barely detectable levels to normal within 12–24 hours. Plasminogen is stable over a wide range of temperatures and pH in plasma and serum. It is a single polypetide chain which, when converted to plasmin, becomes a two-chain molecule connected by a single disulphide bond.

Physiological fibrinolytic activity depends on plasminogen activators in the blood. Increased amounts are found in the plasma after strenuous exercise, emotional stress, surgical operations and other trauma. Plasma activator is difficult to assay because it is extremely labile and in vitro has a half-life of 15 minutes. During clotting plasma activators are absorbed onto fibrin.

Naturally-occurring activators are found in blood, tissue and urine. Tissue activator can be extracted from most human organs with the exception of the placenta. Tissues especially rich in activator include the uterus, ovaries, prostate, heart, lungs, thyroid, adrenal glands and lymph nodes. Activity in tissues is concentrated mainly around blood vessels, veins having greater activity than arteries. Venous occlusion of the limbs will stimulate fibrinolytic activity of the blood and this has been used as a test for evaluating an

9

individual's potential to release activator from the vascular endothelium (Robertson 1971).

Plasmin, the proteolytic enzyme derived from plasminogen can digest many proteins including fibrinogen and fibrin. Normally the action of plasmin is confined to the digestion of fibrin because of the presence of plasmin inhibitors in the blood. Other proteins which can be digested by plasmin include prothrombin, factors V and VIII, glucagon, ACTH and growth hormone.

There are two main inhibitors of the fibrinolytic system: antiactivators which inhibit plasminogen activation and anti-plasmins which are inhibitors of formed plasmin. Antiactivators have been separated (Aoki & Von Kaulla 1971) and identified in human serum (Bennett 1970) and shown to develop during the process of spontaneous blood coagulation (Bennett 1970).

Several aliphatic-amino compounds are competitive inhibitors of plasminogen activation and include epsilon aminocaproic acid (EACA), tranexamic acid (AMCA) and aprotinin (Trasylol) which is commercially prepared from bovine lung.

Both plasma and serum exert a strong inhibitory action on plasmin, and specific antiplasmins have been demonstrated (Bonnar 1975; Bonnar 1978). Platelets have anti-plasmin activity which is probably of importance in stabilising platelet thrombi. Normally plasma antiplasmin levels exceed the levels of plasminogen and hence the levels of potential plasmin.

Fibrin and fibrinogen degradation products (FDP)

When fibrinogen or fibrin is broken down by plasmin, FDP are formed (Fig. 1). Plasmin first splits off fragment X with some smaller fragments A, B and C (Marder 1971). Further digestion of fragment X which is still slowly but completely clottable by thrombin, results in the formation of fragments Y and D, which will not clot under the action of thrombin. Fragment Y is further broken down to fragments D and E, so-called 'end split products'. Fragments X and Y are termed 'high-molecular-weight split products'.

When a fibrin clot is formed approximately 70% of fragment X is retained in the clot, fragment Y is retained to a somewhat lesser extent, and D and E are retained to 10% only.

Serum therefore can contain small amounts of fragment X, larger amounts of Y, D and E, as well as complexes of fibrin monomers, fibrinogen and fragment Y and X. All of these components have

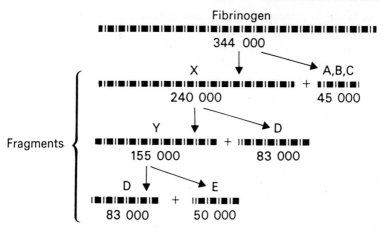

Fig. 1.4 Fibrin degradation products (FDPs) produced by degradation of fibrinogen by plasmin. Molecular weights are shown.

antigenic determinants in common with fibrinogen, and will be recognised by antifibrinogen antisera.

Menstrual blood contains a high level of plasminogen activator which has been correlated with the concentration of activator in the endometrium. Although some workers have been unable to demonstrate fibrinogen or fibrin in menstrual blood (Hahn 1974) and it has been reported that menstrual clots are gels of red cell aggregates (Beller 1971), others have been able to demonstrate fibrin using the electron microscope (Bonnar 1978). The importance of fibrinolysis in menstruation is supported by the decrease in menstrual loss during treatment with the fibrinolytic inhibitor epsilon aminocaproic acid (EACA).

Tests of haemostatic function

There are simple rapid screening tests which establish the competence or otherwise of the haemostatic system. These tests can be performed in any general haematological laboratory and do not require an expert coagulation unit. No attempt is made to give technical details of the tests recommended; these can be found elsewhere (Dacie & Lewis 1975; Ingram et al 1982). It is assumed that this text will be read by clinicians managing patients at the bedside rather than from the laboratory. Emphasis is laid, therefore, on easily available investigations, the results of which will help those in obstetric practice to come to a rapid decision concerning the nature of haemostatic failure in their patients.

Brief reference to additional more complicated tests or those which may be of use in research are to be found in this chapter, or under the relevant subject heading concerning the diagnosis and management of specific conditions associated with defects of haemostasis which can occur in obstetric practice.

Technique of blood collection

All of the tests referred to below are performed on suitably prepared aliquots of specimens of whole blood acquired by venipuncture.

In order to avoid testing artefacts it is essential that the blood is obtained by a quick, efficient, nontraumatic technique, with particular emphasis on the following points:

1. Thromboplastin contamination

Thromboplastin release from damaged tissues may contaminate the specimen and alter the results. This is likely to occur if difficulty is encountered in finding the vein or if the vein is only partly canalised and the flow is slow, or if there is excessive squeezing of tissues and repeated attempts to obtain a specimen with the same needle. In such circumstances the specimen may clot in the tube in spite of the presence of anticoagulant or the coagulation times of the various tests will be altered and not reflect the true situation in vivo. The platelets may aggregate in clumps and give a falsely low count, be it automated or manual (see below).

2. Heparin contamination

Heparin characteristically prolongs the partial thromboplastin time and thrombin time out of proportion to the prothrombin time. As little as 0.05 units of heparin per ml will prolong the coagulation test times (Hathaway & Bonnar 1978). It is customary, though not desirable, to take blood for coagulation tests from lines which have been washed through with fluids containing heparin to keep them patent. My belief is that it is almost impossible to overcome the effect on the blood passing through such a line however much blood is taken and discarded before obtaining a sample for investigation; I would strongly recommend taking blood from another site not previously contaminated with heparin.

3. Fibrinolysis in vitro

Any blood taken into a glass tube without anticoagulant will clot within a few minutes and natural fibrinolysis will continue in vitro. Unless the blood is taken into a fibrinolytic inhibitor such as EACA, a falsely high level of FDPs will be found which bears no relationship to fibrinolysis in vivo. Similarly, leaving a tourniquet on too long before taking the specimen will stimulate local fibrinolytic activity in vivo.

Screening Tests for Haemostatic Function

We are seeking to establish the competence or otherwise of: 1. Vasculature, 2. Coagulation mechanisms, 3. Fibrinolytic system.

1. Tests related to vasculature integrity

a. Bleeding time. The length of time a small skin wound continues to bleed depends largely on the number and function of platelets, i.e. their ability to form plugs at the site of injury. Ivy's method is recommended (Ingram et al 1982) but the test is unpleasant for the patient and tedious if the bleeding is prolonged (normal range up to 7–10 minutes; clearly abnormal — more than 15–20 minutes). It is not of value in assessing haemostatic failure in an obstetric emergency. Its use in coagulation laboratories is mainly in the investigation of bleeding disorders with a normal platelet count (e.g. thrombasthenia Bernard Soulier syndrome, see Ch. 6). It will always be prolonged in the presence of significant thrombocytopenia. Details of platelet function tests can be found elsewhere (Ingram et al 1982).

b. Platelet count. The commonest platelet disorder is thrombocytopenia. It may be an isolated haemostatic defect or part of a generalised consumptive coagulopathy.

The venous blood for examination is taken into commercially provided containers with the anticoagulant EDTA (sequestrene). It is also routinely used when estimation of haemoglobin concentration, haematocrit and white cell count are required. Examination of the blood film by a competent haematology laboratory worker may also

13

provide valuable information concerning the nature of a haemostatic disorder.

In large automated laboratories the count is performed electronically on a diluted whole blood specimen. The platelets are distinguished from other cells in the blood on the basis of size and size distribution. This provides a more accurate assessment of platelet numbers than the visual method performed in small laboratories with less sophisticated machinery. Here anticoagulated blood is diluted in a fluid which lyses red cells and the diluted suspension is counted in a ruled chamber. The platelet count is a valuable rapid screening test in assessing acute obstetric haemostatic failure, particularly in helping the attendants, together with other assessments, to diagnose the presence and severity of disseminated intravascular coagulation (DIC).

The more sophisticated tests which are used in the investigation of autoimmune and alloimmune thrombocytopenia are dealt with under the relevant sections (see Ch. 5).

2. Coagulation mechanisms

Blood for investigation should be taken into trisodium citrate; a measured standard amount of citrate is used so that the dilution factor is constant. It is essential that the exact amount of blood required for laboratory testing is delivered into the citrate-containing bottle or the proportion of anticoagulant to blood will be altered and the results will be unreliable. Variations in haematocrit can introduce similar effects and may have to be allowed for by appropriate adjustments of the proportion of citrate. There are three simple, rapid in vitro tests of the integrity of the coagulation cascade:

a. Partial thromboplastin time (PTT) — intrinsic system. Activated whole blood clotting time.

b. Prothrombin time (PT) — extrinsic system.

c. Thrombin time (TT) — final common pathway.

For the relationship of these tests to the coagulation cascades see Figure 1.5.

Partial thromboplastin time (PTT). This is also known as the PTTK — partial thromboplastin time with kaolin and the activated whole blood clotting time. If normal blood is allowed to clot in a glass tube with no additives the process takes from 4–11 minutes. The time-consuming reactions are those which lead to contact activation and those which cause aggregation and release of phospholipid from platelets. These reactions are accelerated or bypassed by

INTRINSIC SYSTEM   EXTRINSIC SYSTEM

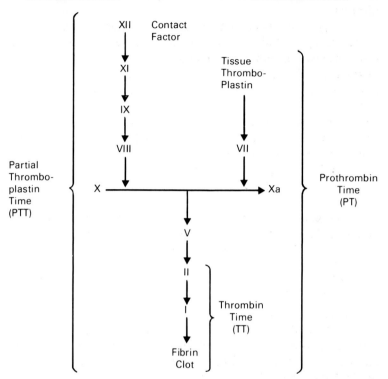

Fig. 1.5 In vitro screening tests of coagulation and their relationship to the systems involved.

preincubation of citrated plasma with kaolin to activate the contact factors and the addition of phospholipid to replace platelet activity.

The measurement of the clotting time of the citrated plasma on addition of calcium and phospholipid under these circumstances gives a crude assessment of the integrity of the intrinsic coagulation system. The normal range usually lies between 35 and 45 s, but all tests must always be compared with a known normal plasma. The time taken to complete this test in the laboratory is a distinct advantage over trying to perform bedside whole clotting tests which provide very little information in an emergency and, in my opinion, are a waste of time (see Ch. 3). The PTT is not only quicker but much more informative. The clotting time is very insensitive and can therefore be dangerously misleading.

Prothrombin time (PT). This test measures the clotting time of citrated plasma after the addition of an optimal concentration of tissue extract (thromboplastin) and recalcification.

Originally introduced by Quick as a measure of prothrombin, factor II, activity. It is now known to depend in addition on reactions between factors V, VII and X and thus is a measure of the overall efficiency of the extrinsic clotting system. Normal range approximately 10–14 s. It has been repeatedly demonstrated (Dacie & Lewis 1975) that the values obtained in any laboratory depend on exactly how the test is undertaken and, in particular, on the source and type of brain thromboplastin used.

For details of the use of the prothrombin time in the control of Warfarin therapy see Chapter 2.

Thrombin time. This test is a measure of the final common pathway of the extrinsic and intrinsic coagulation systems (Fig. 1.5). Thrombin is added to a sample of citrated plasma and the time for a fibrin clot to form is measured. The time taken is affected by the concentration and reaction of fibrin.

Normal plasma will give a thrombin clotting time of 10–15 s. The commonest causes of a delayed thrombin time are the presence of fibrin degradation products, depletion of fibrinogen and the presence of heparin.

Both the clotting time and the appearance of the clot are informative. For further details of the use of this very valuable rapid screening test of haemostatic competence see the section on the investigation of the bleeding obstetric patient (Ch. 3).

Fibrinogen estimation. Fibrinogen titre is a semiquantitative assay of fibrinogen using the thrombin time as a basis for the assay. It is clinically useful and much more rapid than is a chemical estimation of fibrinogen (Dacie & Lewis 1975). Several dilutions of both normal and test plasma samples are clotted with fibrinogen and the highest dilutions in which fibrin clots can be seen are compared.

For further information the tests can be carried out in dilutions of EACA (to prevent fibrinolysis) and protamine sulphate (to overcome the inhibitory effect of FDPs) as well as in saline but for rapidity in an emergency situation direct comparison of the normal and test plasma diluted in saline will give valuable information concerning the amount of functional fibrinogen present in the circulation of the patient.

An even more rapid test for depletion of fibrinogen in obstetric practice has been described (Dacie & Lewis 1975). Using the information that latex particles coated with a rabbit antihumanfibrinogen antisera react with both fibrinogen and fibrin degradation products (see below), if *plasma* samples (not serum) are used failure to agglutinate such particles compared with a normal plasma will indicate gross depletion of fibrinogen in the patient. This test should always be followed by a test for fibrinogen based on its clottability since immunological methods may overestimate the functionally active fibrinogen particularly in the presence of DIC.

Using the above simple tests in the screening of a patient with an acute or chronic haemostatic disorder, together with a detailed clinical history, it is possible to place them into categories or even to make a provisional diagnosis which indicates how to proceed further in order to confirm the provisional diagnosis, e.g. to platelet function tests or individual coagulation factor assays (see Table 1.2).

It is essential that these more exacting tests should be carried out in an expert, competent and specialised laboratory and, because of the rapidity with which changes in coagulation factors take place in vitro, such units usually prefer to see the patient themselves rather than receive blood samples taken at other centres, even if they are delivered by car or other rapid transport.

3. Fibrinolytic system

a. Detection of fibrinogen/fibrin degradation products (FDP). The measurement of the products of plasmin digestion of fibrinogen or fibrin provides an indirect test for fibrinolysis. FDP can be detected in several ways. They interfere with the production of fibrinogen by thrombin and will prolong the thrombin time (see above). Addition of protamine sulphate to plasma containing FDPs will produce fibrin strand formation. Rapid clumping of staphylococci is produced by serum containing FDPs. The most sensitive methods are immunological. Latex particles or red blood cells coated with fibrinogen will be agglutinated on addition of antifibrinogen serum, or particles coated with antibody are agglutinated when mixed with serum or plasma containing fibrinogen or FDP.

The most specific procedure is a two-stage method in which the patient's serum is incubated with antifibrinogen antisera and the residual antibody measured by agglutination of fibrinogen-coated particles. In practice the most rapid assessment of FDPs in the circulation is to add particles coated with fibrinogen antibody (raised in rabbits) to dilutions of the patient's *serum* taken into EACA to prevent in vitro fibrinolysis. In obstetric practice the measurement of

Table 1.2 Results of screening tests in some of the more common haemostatic disorders

	Bleeding time	Platelet count	Partial thromboplastin time	Prothrombin time	Thrombin time
Hereditary					
Factor VIII deficiency Haemophilia A	N	N	↑	N	N
Factor IX deficiency Christmas disease	N	N	↑	N	N
Von Willebrand's disease	↑	N	↑ (or N)	N	N
Thrombasthenia	↑	N	N	N	N
Acquired					
Disseminated intravascular coagulation	↑	↓	↑	↑	↑↑
Idiopathic thrombocytopenia purpura	↑	↓	N	N	N

N = normal

FDPs is usually part of the investigation of suspected acute or chronic DIC. In the acute situation raised FDPs only confirm the presence of DIC, but are not diagnostic and once the specimen is taken the laboratory measurement should be delayed until after the emergency is over so that skilled laboratory workers can be performing a much more valuable service in providing results of coagulation screening tests and blood and blood products suitable for transfusion.

b. Euglobulin clot lysis time (Dacie & Lewis 1975). Plasma is diluted and acidified. A precipitate is formed which contains plasminogen, plasminogen activator and fibrinogen. The precipitate is redissolved; the fibrinogen clotted with thrombin and the time for clot lysis on incubation at 37°C is observed. This is a test of plasminogen activator activity. The normal range is 90 to 240 mins. The test is fiddly, may be difficult to interpret, and requires strict standardisation and precision in the laboratory.

c. Lysis of fibrin plates (Dacie & Lewis 1975[1]). An alternative to this test for the detection of plasminogen activator involves the use of specially prepared fibrin plates. These are inevitably contaminated with plasminogen. If plasminogen activator is present in the test, euglobulin fraction or plasma then lysis of the plate should occur. The area of lysis is proportional to the concentration of plasminogen activator. Again this is a difficult test which is time consuming. The plates are incubated for 24 hours before being read.

d. Assay of plasminogen in plasma (Dacie & Lewis 1975[2]). Streptokinase is added to plasma to convert plasminogen to plasmin and the plasmin activity measured using a spectrophotometric method (normal range 1.5–4 units per ml of plasma). Immunological tests of plasminogen activity have also been described. Low levels occur during systemic fibrinolysis and DIC. Although this test is more rapid than those described above, none of them have any practical place in the management of the obstetric patient with acute haemostatic failure.

The tests described above provide a crude assessment of the competence of haemostatic and fibrinolytic systems.

Any woman who has an inherited or chronic defect of haemostasis which has been identified prior to her index pregnancy should be delivered in a unit which has immediate access to expert investigation, advice and supportive therapy (see Chs. 5 and 6).

If a woman develops such a problem during pregnancy, e.g. factor VIII inhibitor or thrombocytopenia, it would be wise to transfer her to such a unit if there is time.

Specific problems appertaining to management of thrombocytopenia, carriers of haemophilia, etc. will be dealt with under the relevant chapter headings (Chs. 5 and 6).

Haemostatic mechanisms during normal pregnancy

Platelets during pregnancy

Number size and function

There have been a number of conflicting reports concerning the platelet count and platelet function of normal pregnancy. One of the difficulties has been the definition of normal pregnancy. Most investigators agree that low grade chronic intravascular coagulation within the uteroplacental circulation is a part of the physiological response of all women to pregnancy (see below). This is partially compensated and it is not surprising therefore that the platelets should be involved at some level. The degree of compensation which is variable will determine whether the platelet count differs from the normal nonpregnant state and this is the parameter of platelet function which has been most widely studied in pregnancy (Bonnar 1981). Eleven reports of platelet count during normal pregnancy (Sejeny et al 1975) varied appreciably in their findings. The numbers in the series were small and the counts were performed manually. The introduction of automated platelet counters has facilitated the investigation of larger numbers. However, there is still some variation of findings in published reports (Pitkin & Witte 1979). A special study of 44 normal pregnancies using an automated platelet counter showed no significant change compared with the normal nonpregnant state (Fenton et al 1977). Others have reported a significant decrease in the numbers of circulating platelets as pregnancy advances (O'Brien 1976). A recent large study (Fay et al 1983) showed that in the 2066 women studied there was a significant fall in the platelet count during the last eight weeks of pregnancy, but the platelet count was still well within the normal nonpregnant range in every case. This same study showed a significant rise in the mean platelet volume during the last four weeks of pregnancy.

As young platelets are large and become progressively smaller with age, the authors took the finding of increasing platelet volume, together with decreasing platelet count, to support the concept of platelet hyperdestruction during pregnancy as part of the process of chronic intravascular coagulation of normal pregnancy, which progressively increases towards term (McKay 1981).

However, other studies have shown no significant difference in platelet lifespan between nonpregnant and healthy pregnant women (Rakoczi et al 1979; Wallenburg & Von Kessel 1978), although significant differences are found in pre-eclampsia and pregnancies complicated by intra-uterine growth retardation (IUGR) without evidence of pre-eclampsia (Redman et al 1978) (see Ch. 4).

There are very few convincing published studies of platelet function during normal pregnancy. Two studies performed more than 15 years ago showed no significant difference in platelet adhesiveness during healthy pregnancy from the normal non-pregnant state (McKay et al 1964; Shaper et al 1968) although there was a marked increase in platelet adhesiveness in the immediate postpartum period (Shaper et al 1968). For changes in platelet function observed in the course of pre-eclampsia and pregnancies complication by fetal growth impairment see Chapter 4.

A more recent study (Lewis et al 1980) demonstrated significantly more aggregable platelets in a small number of women during late pregnancy and the puerperium compared with nonpregnant controls.

Prostacyclin in pregnancy

The concentration of $6-OXO-PGF_{1\alpha}$, the stable hydration product of prostacyclin (PGI_2), probably reflects the circulating concentration of active PGI_2. This has been measured in a small number of women during early, mid- and late pregnancy and in the first week after delivery. The levels of $6-OXO-PGF_{1\alpha}$ were found to be double those in nonpregnant women on analysis of blood taken during late pregnancy and the puerperium (Lewis et al 1980). The source of the increase in prostacyclin is not known but Lewis & colleagues (1980) suggest that it could be derived from the placenta and uterus, since both are known to generate prostacyclin in vitro (Myatt & Elder 1977; Omini et al 1979). High concentrations of $6-OXO-PGF_{1\alpha}$ have also been detected in amniotic fluid (Mitchell et al 1979).

Another study has shown that during early normal pregnancy the plasmatic activity of prostacyclin stimulating factor was similar to that in nonpregnant women but that in late pregnancy the activity was significantly depressed (Remuzzi et al 1981). Previously Remuzzi & colleagues (1979) had shown that prostacyclin activity increased during late normal pregnancy. They suggest that possibly the activity of prostacyclin stimulating factor is depressed in late normal pregnancy by a feedback mechanism.

Neonatal production of prostacyclin has also been measured using umbilical vessels obtained at birth (Stuart et al 1981, Mäkilä et al 1983; Downing et al 1982). The source of the normal increase in circulating prostacyclin in maternal circulation in pregnancy is not clear, PGI_2 could be derived from the uterus, the placenta, or the fetus, which all appear to have vascular elements actively synthesising the substance. Increased prostacyclin production may be involved with the characteristic vasodilation which occurs in pregnancy. It may be an adaptive response to a primary increase in platelet aggregability (Lewis et al 1980).

Recently Mäkilä & colleagues (1983) have shown a clear relationship between prostacyclin production by the umbilical artery and blood flow in the fetus; pregnancies complicated by placental insufficiency showing reduced prostacyclin production in the umbilical artery.

For further discussion of the possible role of prostacyclin in the pathogenesis and management of pre-eclampsia and intrauterine growth impairment, see Chapter 4.

Coagulation system

Normal pregnancy is accompanied by major changes in the coagulation system, with increases in the levels of factors VII, VIII, and X and a particularly marked increase in the level of plasma fibrinogen (Fig.1.4). The increased quantity of fibrinogen in the plasma alters the negative surface charge of the red cells which, on standing, will form aggregates in a pattern described as *rouleaux*, which settle in a glass tube more quickly than single erythrocytes. The increase in fibrinogen is probably the chief cause of the accelerated erthrocyte sedimentation rate observed during pregnancy (Wintrobe 1974).

The effect of pregnancy on the coagulation factors can be detected from about the third month of gestation. The plasma fibrinogen level increases from nonpregnant levels of about 2.5–4.0 g/l to as high as 6.0 g/l during late pregnancy and labour. If the increase of plasma volume is taken into consideration the amount of circulating fibrinogen during late pregnancy is at least double that of the nonpregnant state. This marked rise in fibrinogen results from increased synthesis as has been shown in pregnant monkeys (Bonnar

1978). The elevation of factor VII during pregnancy may be increased as much as tenfold; an increase in this factor has also been observed in women taking oestrogen/progestogen contraceptives (Gjonnaesse 1973).

Factor VIII, antihaemophilic factor, is elevated during late pregnancy, the coagulation activity being approximately twice that in the nonpregnant state. Some workers have found a parallel increase both in the biological activity of factor VIII and in the factor VIII-related antigen (Bennett & Ratnoff 1972), while others have found an increase in the ratio between the antigenic and coagulant activity (Bouma et al 1973; Van Royen & Tengate 1973).

Elevations of factor IX (Christmas factor) during pregnancy have been reported by several authors, as have decreases in factor XI, with levels down to 60–70% of the nonpregnant value (Bonnar 1978). An increase in factor XII and a decrease in antithrombin III have been described (Van Royen & Tengate 1973), as well as a gradual fall in fibrin stabilising factor reaching 50% of the normal nonpregnant value at term (Coopland et al 1969).

Increased concentrations of high-molecular-weight fibrin/fibrinogen complexes in the plasma have been demonstrated during normal pregnancy (Fletcher & Alkjaersig 1973) and confirmed more recently by comparing the levels in normal pregnancy with those found in nonpregnant age-matched controls (McKillop et al 1976). An increase in the level of fibrinopeptide A and a thrombin-like influence on factor V activity has also been described (Van Royen 1974).

Fletcher & colleagues (1979) studied fibrinogen catabolism in 27 patients from early pregnancy through delivery and up to 4 months postpartum using a noninvasive technique of plasma fibrinogen chromatography. High-molecular-weight fibrinogen or fibrinogen/fibrin complexes were measured as an indicator of fibrin function in vivo. During the second gestational month high-molecular-weight fibrinogen/fibrin complexes were significantly raised and this preceded the rise in plasma fibrinogen. These results suggest that intravascular fibrin deposition is the earliest and most persistent alteration in blood coagulation function during pregnancy.

There appears to be an increased ability to neutralise heparin during late pregnancy as demonstrated by the need for a moderately increased dose to maintain constant plasma levels in those women receiving prophylactic low-dose heparin during the third trimester (Bonnar 1976).

These changes in the coagulation system during normal pregnancy

23

are consistent with a continuing low grade process of coagulant activity. Using electron microscopy, fibrin deposition can be demonstrated in the intervillous space of the placenta and in the walls of spiral arteries supplying the placenta (Sheppard & Bonnar 1974). As pregnancy advances, the elastic lamina and smooth muscle of these spiral arteries are replaced by a matrix containing fibrin. This allows an expansion of the lumen to accommodate an increasing blood flow and reduces the pressure in arterial blood flowing to the placenta. At placental separation during normal childbirth, a blood flow of 500–800 ml per minute has to be staunched within seconds or serious haemorrhage will occur. Myometrial contraction plays a vital role in securing haemostasis by reducing the blood flow to the placental site. At separation of the placenta, rapid closure of the terminal part of the spiral arteries by the unique mechanism of myometrial contraction will be facilitated by the structural changes described (Bonnar 1978). The placental site is rapidly covered by a fibrin mesh following delivery: the amount of fibrinogen deposited represents 5–10% of the total circulating fibrinogen.

The increased levels of fibrinogen and coagulation factors during pregnancy probably represent a compensatory response to local utilisation. The resulting hypercoagulability will be advantageous to meet the sudden demand for haemostatic components at placental separation (Howie 1979).

Fibrinolysis

Plasma fibrinolytic activity is decreased during pregnancy, remains low during labour and delivery and returns to normal within one hour of placental delivery (Bonnar et al 1969). Fibrinolytic activity in the walls of veins is reduced during late pregnancy (Astedt 1972).

The rapid return of systemic fibrinolytic activity to normal following delivery of the placenta together with the fact that the placenta has been shown to contain inhibitors which block fibrinolysis (Uszynski & Abildgard 1971) suggests that inhibition of fibrinolysis during pregnancy is mediated through the placenta.

Since fibrinolysis is depressed during pregnancy, the level of FDP will not necessarily reflect the amount of local intravascular coagulation (Bonnar 1978).

The existence of any impairment of fibrinolysis during normal pregnancy has been questioned (Fletcher et al 1979). It has been suggested that the low levels of plasminogen activator in the plasma are the result of absorption of plasminogen activator to fibrin and that the fivefold increase in fibrin deposition compared with the normal nonpregnant state is accompanied by significant increase in compensatory fibrinolysis.

The increase of FDP in the circulation during labour (Uszynski & Abildgard 1971; Bonnar 1978) may originate from the uterus. FDP levels in uterine blood during caesarean section carried out in the course of labour were considerably higher than those during elective caesarean section (Hahn 1974).

Haemostatic problems associated with pregnancy

As has already been outlined, pregnancy is known to induce complex changes in the physiological systems concerned with haemostasis. The alterations in the coagulation and fibrinolytic systems which take place during pregnancy, together with the increased blood volume and unique phenomenon of myometrial contraction, help to combat the hazard of haemorrhage during and after placental separation; however they carry the risk of more rapid and increased response to coagulant stimuli. The characteristic tendency to venous stasis in the lower limbs may provide initiating conditions and the incidence of venous thrombosis, though low, is undoubtedly raised during pregnancy.

The most recent Report on Confidential Enquiries into Maternal Deaths in England and Wales (1982) reports that pulmonary embolism has become the major single cause of maternal mortality in the triennium 1976–1978.

The local activation of the clotting system during parturition (Kleiner et al 1970; Bonnar et al 1970) carries with it a risk not only of thrombo-embolism but of disseminated intravascular coagulation, consumption of clotting factors and platelets leading to severe generalised — and in particular uterine — bleeding. Despite the advances in obstetric care and highly-developed blood transfusion services, haemorrhage still constitutes a major factor in maternal mortality and morbidity.

Thus far, an account of the physiology of normal haemostasis and the changes in haemostatic mechanisms during normal pregnancy has been given. This is intended to serve as a basis for understanding and managing disorders in obstetrics associated with derangements of the coagulation and fibrinolytic systems.

Coagulation Problems During Pregnancy

REFERERCES

Aoki N, Von Kaulla K V 1971 Human serum plasminogen anti-activator: its distinction from anti-plasmin. American Journal of Physiology 220: 1137–1145

Astedt B 1972 On fibrinolysis. Acta obstetricia et gynecologica Scandinavica 51: (suppl 18) 1–45

Beller F K 1971 Observations on the clotting of menstrual blood and clot formation. American Journal of Obstetrics and Gyncecology III: 535–546

Bennett N B 1970 Further studies on an inhibitor of plasminogen activation: release of inhibitor during coagulation and thrombus formation. Thrombosis et diathesis haemorrhagica 23: 553–561

Bennett B, Ratnoff OD 1972 Changes in AHF procoagulant activity and AHF-like antigen in normal pregnancy and following exercise and pneumoencephalography. Journal of Laboratory and Clinical Medicine 80: 256–263

Biggs R, Denson K W E, Akman N, Borrett R, Haddon M E 1970 Antithrombin III, Antifactor Xa and heparin. British Journal of Haematology 19: 283–305

Bloom A L, Thomas P P (eds) 1981 Haemostasis and Thrombosis; Churchill Livingstone, Edinburgh

Bonnar J 1975 The blood coagulation and fibrinolytic systems during pregnancy. Clinics in Obstetrics and Gynaecology 2: 321–344

Bonnar J 1976 Long term self-administered heparin therapy for prevention and treatment of thrombo-embolic complications in pregnancy. In: Kakkar V J, Thomas D P (eds) Heparin chemistry and clinical usage, Academic Press, New York, p 247–260

Bonnar J 1978 Haemostasis in pregnancy and coagulation disorders. In: Scientific basis of obstetrics and gynaecology, 2nd edn. Churchill Livingstone, Edinburgh, p 250–273

Bonnar J 1981 Haemostasis and coagulation disorders in pregnancy. In: Bloom A. L, Thomas D P (eds) Haemostasis and thrombosis. Churchill Livingstone, Edinburgh, p 454–471

Bonnar J, McNicol G P, Douglass A S 1969 Fibrinolytic enzyme system and pregnancy. British Medical Journal iii: 387–389

Bonnar J, Prentice C R M, McNicol G P, Douglas A S 1970 Haemostatic mechanism in uterine circulation during placental separation. British Medical Journal ii: 564–567

Bouma B N, Sixma J J, Mouik J A Van, Mochtar I A 1973 Immunological determination of antihaemophilic factor A (factor VIII). Netherlands Journal of Medicine 16: 54

Coopland A, Alkjaersig N, Fletcher A P 1969 Reduction in plasma factor XIII (fibrin stabilising factor) concentration during pregnancy. Journal of Laboratory and Clinical Medicine 73: 144–153

Dacie J V, Lewis S M 1975 Practical haematology, 5th edn, Churchill Livingstone, Edinburgh, p 369[1], 570[2]

Department of Health and Social Security 1982 Report on Confidential Enquiries into Maternal Deaths in England and Wales 1976–1978. DHSS 26. Her Majesty's Stationery Office, London

Downing I, Shepherd G L, Lewis J P 1982 Kinetics of prostacyclin synthetase in umbilical artery microsomes from normal and pre-eclamptic pregnancies. British Journal of Pharmacology 13: 195–198

Fay R A, Hughes A O, Farron N T 1983 Platelets in pregnancy: hyperdestruction in pregnancy. Obstetrics and Gynecology 61: 238–240

Fenton V, Saunders K, Gavill I 1977 The platelet count in pregnancy. Journal of Clinical Pathology 30: 68–69

Fletcher A P, Alkjaersig N 1973 Laboratory diagnosis of intravascular coagulation. In: Poller L (ed) Recent advances in thrombosis. Churchill Livingstone, Edinburgh, p 87–111

Fletcher A P, Alkjaersig N K, Burstein R 1979 The influence of pregnancy upon blood coagulation and plasma fibrinolytic enzyme function. American Journal of Obstetrics and Gynecology 134: 743–751

Gaffney P J 1981 The fibrinolytic system. In: Bloom A L, Thomas D P (eds) Haemostasis and thrombosis, Churchill Livingstone, Edinburgh, pp 198–224

Gjonnaesse H 1973 Cold-promoted activation of factor VII. Gynecological Investigation 4: 61–72

Hahn L 1974 Fibrinogen-fibrin degradation products in uterine and peripheral blood during caesarean section. Acta obstetricia et gynecologica scandinavica 53: (supp 28) 1–7

Hardisty R M 1982 Platelets, blood vessels and haemostasis: disorders of platelet and vascular function: In: Hardisty R M, Weatherall D J (eds) Blood and its disorders, Blackwell Scientific Publications, Oxford, pp 1031–1074

Howie P W 1979 Blood clotting and fibrinolysis in pregnancy. Postgraduate Medical Journal 55: 363–366

Ingram G I C, Brozovic M, Slater N G P 1982 Haemostatic mechanisms. In: Bleeding disorders. Investigation and management, 2nd edn. Blackwell Scientific Publications, Oxford

Kleiner G J, Merskey C, Johnson A J, Markus W D 1970 Defibrination in normal and abnormal parturition. British Journal of Haematology 19: 159–178

Lewis J P, Boylan P, Friedman L A, Hensby C N, Downing I 1980 Prostacyclin in pregnancy. British Medical Journal 280: 1581–1582

Macfarlane R G 1964 An enzyme cascade in the blood clotting mechanism and its function as a biochemical amplifier. Nature 202: 494–499

McKay D G 1981 Chronic intravascular coagulation in normal pregnancy and pre-eclampsia. Contributions to Nephrology 25: 108–119

McKay D G, De Bacalao E B, Sedlis A 1964 Platelet adhesiveness in toxaemia of pregnancy. American Journal of Obstetrics and Gynecology 90: 1315–1318

McKillop C, Howie P W, Forbes C D, Prentice C R M 1976 Soluble fibrinogen/fibrin complexes in pre-eclampsia. Lancet i: 56–58

Mäkilä U-M, Jouppila P, Kirkinen P, Viinikka L, Ulikorkala O 1983 Relation between umbilical prostacyclin production and blood-flow in the fetus. Lancet i: 728–729

Marder V J 1971 Identification and purification of fibrin degradation products produced by plasmin: Considerations on the structure of fibrinogen. Scandinavian Journal of Haematology (Suppl.13) 21–36

Mitchell M D, Keirse M J N C, Brunt J D, Anderson A B M, Turnbull A C 1979 Concentrations of the prostacyclin metabolite 6 keto-prostaglandin $F_{1\alpha}$ in amniotic fluid during late pregnancy and labour. British Journal of Obstetrics and Gynaecology 86: 350–353

Moncada M D, Vane J R 1979 Arachidonic acid metabolites and the interactions between platelets and blood-vessel walls. New England Journal of Medicine 300: 1142–1147

Moncada S, Gryglewski R J, Bunting S, Vane J H 1976 An enzyme isolated from arteries transforms prostaglandin endoperoxides to an unstable substance that inhibits platelet aggregation. Nature 263: 663–665

Moncada S, Vane J R 1978 Pharmacology and endogenous roles of prostaglandin endoperoxides, thromboxane A_2 and prostacyclin. Pharmacological Reviews 30: 293–331

Moncada S, Vane J R 1981 Prostacyclin: Haemostatic regulator or biological curiosity? Clinical Science 61: 369–372

Myatt L, Elder M G 1977 Inhibition of platelet aggregation by a placental substance with prostacyclin-like activity. Nature 268: 159–160

Niewarowski S 1981 Platelet release reaction and secreted platelet proteins. In:

27

Bloom A L, Thomas D P, Haemostasis and thrombosis, Churchill Livingstone, Edinburgh, pp 73–83

O'Brien J R 1976 Platelet counts in normal pregnancy. Journal of Clinical Pathology 29: 174

Omini C, Folco G C, Pasargiklian R, Fano M, Berti F 1979 Prostacyclin (PGI$_2$) in pregnant human uterus. Prostaglandins 17: 113–120

Pitkin R M, Witte D L 1979 Platelet and leukocyte counts in pregnancy. Journal of the American Medical Association 242: 2696–2698

Rakoczi I, Tallian F, Bagdany S, Gati I 1979 Platelet lifespan in normal pregnancy and pre-eclampsia as determined by a nonradioisotope technique. Thrombosis Research 15: 553–556

Redman C W G, Bonnar J, Beilin C J 1978 Early platelet consumption in pre-eclampsia. British Medical Journal i: 467–469

Remuzzi G et al 1978 Haemolytic uraemic syndrome; deficiency of plasma factor(s) regulating prostacyclin activity. Lancet ii: 871–872

Remuzzi G et al 1979 Prostacyclin and human fetal circulation. Prostaglandins 18: 341–348

Remuzzi G, et al 1981 Plasmatic regulation of vascular prostacyclin in pregnancy. British Medical Journal 282: 512–514

Robertson B 1971 On thrombosis, thrombolysis and fibrinolysis. Acta chirurgica scandinavica (1972) suppl. no. 421, p 1–51

Sejeny S A, Eastham R D, Baker S R 1975 Platelet counts during normal pregnancy. Journal of Clinical Pathology, 28: 812–813

Shaper A G, Kear J, Macintosh D M, Kyobe J, Njama D 1968 The platelet count, platelet adhesiveness and aggregation and the mechanism of fibrinolytic inhibition in pregnancy and the puerperium. Journal of Obstetrics and Gynaecology of the British Commonwealth 75: 433–441

Sheppard B L, Bonnar J 1974 The ultrastructure of the arterial supply of the human placenta in early and late pregnancy. Journal of Obstetrics and Gynaecology of the British Commonwealth 81: 497–511

Stuart M J et al 1981 Decreased prostacyclin production! A characteristic of chronic placental insufficiency syndromes. Lancet i: 1126–1128

Uszynski M, Abildgard U 1971 Separation and characterisation of two fibrinolytic inhibitors from human placenta. Thrombosis et diathesis haemorrhagica 25: 580–589

Van Royen E A 1974 Haemostasis in human pregnancy and delivery. MD Thesis, University of Amsterdam

Van Royen E A, Tengate J W 1973 Antigen-biological activity ratio for factor VIII in late pregnancy. Lancet 11: 449–450

Vane J R 1971 Inhibition of prostaglandin synthesis as a mechanism of action for aspirin-like drugs. Nature (New Biology) 231: 232–235

Wallenburg H C S, Van Kessel 1978 Platelet lifespan in normal pregnancy as determined by a nonradio-isotopic technique. British Journal of Obstetrics and Gynecology 85: 33–36

Wintrobe M M 1974 Clinical haematology, 7th edn. Lea & Febiger, Philadephia, p 126

2

Thrombo-embolism during pregnancy

Incidence and significance

The profound changes in the haemostatic mechanism during pregnancy (see Ch. 1), together with some suppression of fibrinolysis, result in an overall increase in coagulation factors, particularly fibrinogen. These changes, together with the increased total blood volume help to combat the hazard of haemorrhage at delivery, but carry with them an increased risk of thrombo-embolism. Pulmonary embolism, the second most frequent cause of maternal mortality since 1955, has now become the major single cause of maternal death associated with pregnancy. In the triennium 1976–78, 47 deaths were coded to pulmonary embolism, approximately one-third occurring in the antenatal period (DHSS 1982).

Incidence antenatal and postnatal

The number of maternal deaths overall during pregnancy and the puerperium over the past 50 years have decreased dramatically even when those due to abortion are excluded. The Report on Confidential Enquiries into Maternal Deaths in England and Wales (DHSS 1982) shows that the total number of deaths has fallen steadily apart from a small increase in postpartum embolism in the triennium 1976–78, but the proportion occurring in the antenatal period has increased sharply. Thrombo-embolism was previously regarded as a complication of the puerperium. Only 4 of the 138 women in the 1952–54 period died during pregnancy, but since 1961 25% of the deaths have occurred during the antenatal period and have been distributed throughout the 40 weeks gestation period. In the period 1970–72 one third of the deaths, and in the period 1972–75 14 of the 35 deaths, occurred in the antenatal period. The most recent Confidential Enquiries published in 1982, covering the period 1976–78 shows, for the first time, an overall increase in total numbers of fatal pulmonary embolism, 14 of the total of 47 occurring in the antenatal period (DHSS 1982).

Predisposing factors to thrombo-embolism associated with pregancy are age, parity, obesity, caesarean section and other operative forms of delivery and oestrogen treatment to suppress lactation. The decline in mortality from pulmonary embolism in the puerperium could be attributed to a number of factors: the trend towards younger mothers and smaller families; the virtual disappearance of traumatic operative delivery hence early ambulation, and better diagnosis and treatment. Obstetricians are aware of the risk of oestrogen treatment for suppression of lactation and do not advise it. On the other hand the rise in the proportion of deaths during the antenatal period could be the result of the increased hospital admission and subsequent bed rest for complications of pregnancy such as mild hypertension and antepartum haemorrhage. The figures from the Confidential Enquiries also show that the total number of deaths following all forms of vaginal delivery has fallen steadily, whereas the number following caesarean section has not fallen so dramatically, but the proportion of women delivered by caesarean section in the last 20 years has greatly increased and now represents over 7.0% of all deliveries making those delivering vaginally a selected group. An increase in the proportion of caesarean sections in the total number of deliveries from 5.3% in 1973 to 7.6% in 1978 is reported (DHSS 1982). It is difficult to obtain accurate data for nonfatal deep vein thrombosis and pulmonary embolism, because these conditions are not easy to diagnose and present particular problems of diagnosis in pregnancy (see below). An incidence of deep vein thrombosis of 0.18% in 25 082 pregnancies at the Mayo Clinic has been reported (Aaro & Juergens 1971).

At Queen Charlotte's there have been 20 cases of deep vein thrombosis and 10 cases of pulmonary embolism associated with about 35 000 deliveries between 1970 and 1980, an overall incidence of 0.09 per cent. Confirmation of these diagnoses were obtained by venogram or by scan in the majority of cases (de Swiet et al 1981).

We are faced therefore with the difficult problem of managing a condition which occurs rarely during pregnancy, but which is a major cause of maternal mortality.

Diagnosis

Deep vein thrombosis

The history and physical signs of this condition are described in standard medical text books, but it is clear that it is very difficult to make an accurate diagnosis based on physical signs alone (Simpson et al 1980). Women who do not have a typical history are unlikely to have a deep vein thrombosis but this hypothesis has not been tested. There are several noninvasive investigations available (Browse 1976) which include:

1. Beta-thromboglobulin estimation as an indication of blood-clotting in vivo.

2. Doppler blood measurement flow.

3. Impedance plethysmography which detects reduced blood flow in the femoral vein of the affected limb.

4. ^{131}I-labelled fibrinogen uptake which demonstrates the blood clot.

5. Venography.

The standard screening investigation is to measure the uptake of ^{131}I-labelled fibrinogen. However, radioactive iodine should not be used in pregnancy. In the antenatal period the free label is trapped by the fetal thyroid and can cause hypothyroidism (Exis & Graeme 1974) and subsequent carcinoma. It is secreted in high concentration in the breast milk and the same risks therefore apply to the breast-fed infant. None of the diagnostic techniques at present available outside the specialised vascular laboratory approaches the precision of venography, although it is possible that subsequent modification or combinations of techniques will do so (Flanigan et al 1978; Hull et al 1977). Because of the hazards of treatment to the mother and particularly the fetus in the index and future pregnancies (see below), a suspected deep vein thrombosis should be confirmed by venography in all patients unless the clinical diagnosis seems overwhelmingly certain: for example, in severe proximal iliac vein thrombosis where the whole limb is markedly swollen. Venography of the femoral and more distal veins can be performed in pregnancy with relative safety if there is adequate shielding of the uterus. The direct radiation dose is very small although there will be some additional scattered radiation.

Phlebography remains the reference method both in research and for routine purposes for establishing the presence or absence of deep venous thrombosis. The clinical impression has always been that phlebography is harmless. However, a disquieting report (Albrechtsson & Olsson 1976) suggested that thrombosis and embolism may be caused by phlebography. Later studies confirmed this report but showed clearly that postphlebography thrombosis was only associated with the extensively used hypertonic contrast media. If these were replaced by the newer isotonic medium metrinamide (Amupaque) there appeared to be no postinvestigation incidence of venous thrombo-embolism (Laerum et al 1980). Also if a patient is already effectively anticoagulated the risk of DVT after phlebography with hypertonic contrast media is reduced. This is often the case during pregnancy when confirmation of a clinically suspected DVT is sought before continuing long-term anticoagulants. It has been suggested that any patient not on oral anticoagulant therapy should be given heparin when they are undergoing phlebography with hypertonic contrast media (Laerum et al 1980). Metrinamide has additional advantages: it causes less pain and less local reaction but it is considerably more expensive than hypertonic contrast media. My opinion is that the hazard of thrombosis following phlebography has been greatly exaggerated and there is no adequate alternative for the diagnosis of DVT. Certainly the hazards of long-term anticoagulation during pregnancy and the puerperium far outweigh the very small risk of inducing a DVT.

Pulmonary embolus

The diagnosis of major pulmonary embolus is not often in doubt, but major pulmonary embolus is often preceded by smaller emboli. A high index of clinical suspicion is essential to diagnose these. The characteristic physical signs are well described in the standard text books. It should be emphasised however that the electrocardiograph may be normal or may show abnormal features (S_1, Q_3, T_3) which are associated with pregnancy alone rather than with pulmonary embolus (de Swiet et al 1981). Since it is important to make an accurate diagnosis of thrombo-embolism during pregnancy before hazardous and perhaps unnecessary therapy is embarked upon, lung scans with ventilation perfusion imaging should be undertaken in all suspected cases. The isotopes used in these scans, [81]krypton[m] for ventilation and [99]technetium[m] for perfusion have very short half-lives and the radiation to the fetus is minimal.

Management of thrombo-embolism during pregnancy

Surgery

Patients who have a life-threatening reduction in cardiac output following pulmonary embolus should be transferred to a cardiothoracic centre and undergo embolectomy under cardio-pulmonary bypass. Patients who have massive iliofemoral thrombosis should also be transferred to such a unit in case they require urgent surgical intervention.

Defibrinating and fibrinolytic agents

A high incidence of fetal death associated with haemorrhage of the placental site was found in the mouse and rabbit using Ancrod (Arvin) the purified fraction of the venom of the Malayan pit viper (Penn et al 1971). This should not be given in human pregnancy.

The administration of streptokinase and urokinase can result in severe haemorrhage from the placental site if administered when delivery is imminent or within the first postpartum week. In view of this hazard streptokinase and urokinase are not recommended except where surgical intervention is not possible, the risk of severe haemorrhage is accepted and prepared for and where fatal pulmonary embolism appears likely (Bonnar 1981a).

Anticoagulants and laboratory control of their use

Anticoagulant therapy is used to prevent the occurrence of thrombosis or the further propagation of an existing thrombus.

Anticoagulant drugs have little effect upon an established thrombus. The dissolution of the thrombus is left to the stimulated natural fibrinolytic processes of the body. In some situations, defibrinating and fibrinolytic agents may be used to speed the process but their use during pregnancy is hazardous and rarely if ever indicated (see above).

There are two main classes of anticoagulant drugs which are commonly used in association with pregnancy:

1. The orally administered coumarin derivatives and indanediones, which act by interfering with the synthesis in the liver of vitamin K-

dependent factors, factors II, VII, IX and X. Warfarin, a coumarin derivative, has emerged over the last decade as the oral anticoagulant used in clinical practice almost exclusively. Indanediones, particularly phenindione have unacceptable side effects.

2. Heparin and heparinoids which have a complex action on clotting: the two main effects are interference with conversion of fibrinogen to fibrin by thrombin and an inhibition of activation of factor X → factor Xa at a key position linking the intrinsic and extrinsic coagulation pathways (see Figs 1.2, 1.5).

Warfarin

The advantage of warfarin is that it can be taken by mouth but its main disadvantages during pregnancy are that:

1. It crosses the placenta (molecular weight 1000), and has adverse effects on the fetus throughout the antenatal period (see below). These include teratogenicity in the first trimester and an increasing haemorrhagic hazard to term, maximal during labour and delivery.

2. A woman who is adequately anticoagulated on warfarin can bleed disastrously if an obstetric complication such as premature placental separation occurs or if urgent caesarean section or instrumental delivery has to be performed.

3. It has a prolonged effect and the action cannot be reversed rapidly although administration of vitamin K will achieve reversal within 24 hours. The only rapid method of reversing the effect is by infusion with fresh frozen plasma to restore the depleted coagulation factors.

4. Because of the elevated clotting factors in pregnancy (see Ch. 1) and the increasing plasma volume, the requirements during pregnancy are changing constantly and much more frequent monitoring and control of dosage is necessary, than during the nonpregnant state.

5. Drugs that interact with warfarin make its control more difficult and may increase the risk of bleeding in the mother and fetus. In particular, antibiotics commonly used in the treatment of urinary tract infection will alter dramatically the requirements of warfarin. If the previously therapeutic dose is continued in the face of antibiotic treatment, dangerously low levels of coagulation factors or inadequate anticoagulation can result.

Laboratory control of warfarin

The purpose of laboratory control is to achieve and maintain a level of hypocoagulability which is effective in preventing thrombosis, but is not sufficient to make the risk of spontaneous haemorrhage appreciable. It is not realistic or in fact possible to induce a derangement of normal haemostatic mechanisms without accepting some risk of bleeding.

Thrombotest of Owren (Dacie & Lewis 1975) measures overall clotting activity and the result is influenced by deficiencies of all of the vitamin K-dependent factors, i.e. II, VII, IX and X. The thrombotest is a very satisfactory alternative test for anticoagulant clinics. It can be performed on capillary blood or on uncentrifuged venous whole blood which facilitates a speedy result obtained while the patient is waiting. The commercial thrombotest reagent is available world-wide so that the thrombotest value has international appreciation.

Prothrombin time. Of the methods available for the laboratory control of warfarin therapy the prothrombin time of Quick is the most popular in the United Kingdom (Dacie & Lewis 1975). This test is basically an examination of the integrity of the extrinsic coagulation pathway (see Figs 1.2, 1.5) but as such is also a crude assay of the vitamin K-dependent factors II, VII and X (with the exception of factor IX).

In the United Kingdom I would recommend the use of prothrombin time for warfarin anticoagulant control during pregnancy and the puerperium; there is strict quality control of this method using the British Comparative Thromboplastin. In the United Kingdom the standard British Comparative Thromboplastin (BCT) was introduced in 1969 with a system of reporting the prothrombin time termed the British Ratio. The BCT reference reagent or its mass produced counterpart, the Manchester Comparative Reagent (MCR) are used in most United Kingdom hospitals for routine work.

This means that in a laboratory attached to a maternity unit which performs relatively few tests such as our own, there will be accuracy and precision compared with laboratories dealing with hundreds of specimens, assuming there is participation in the quality control programme. Also, should urgent investigation be required at any time at another laboratory the coagulation status can be quickly assessed especially if the woman concerned carries an anticoagulant card with current dosage of warfarin and the most recent prothrombin time recorded.

This estimation is performed on citrated plasma and can be undertaken while the woman waits, if she is not an inpatient. The current recommended therapeutic level gives a prothrombin time of 2.0–4.0 times greater than that of the normal control plasma. This is rather higher than the previously recommended prothrombin ratio of 1.7 to 3.0 for prophylaxis. However a less rigorous regime, with a ratio of 2.0 to 2.5 has been shown to be equally effective (Taberner et al 1978) and this is the recommended ratio during pregnancy in order to protect the fetus.

One problem not clearly dealt with in most practical text books is how to arrive at the initial safe-maintenance dose of warfarin. The difficulty arises because there is a delay of approximately 24–48 hours between the initial dose and any significant detectable change in the prothrombin time. This depends on the half-life of the coagulation factors affected by warfarin. If warfarin therapy follows subcutaneous heparin (see below) then it is recommended that heparin be continued for 36 hours (3 injections) after the first oral dose of warfarin has been given. Poller (1981) suggests:

Initial dose of warfarin 20–30 mg	1st day	
10 mg	2nd day	
1–25 mg	maintenance dose	

It is common practice to attempt a rapid effect of oral anticoagulant therapy by giving a loading dose. The larger the initial dose, the more dramatic the prolongation of the prothrombin time at the 24–48 hour period.

There is no doubt that in situations where prophylaxis alone is required (unusual with warfarin during pregnancy) then the use of a loading dose is difficult to justify. However, in practice at Queen Charlotte's Maternity Hospital, London, we have found the following regime to work very well, although I cannot justify it scientifically!

Day 1	any time	30 mg warfarin
Day 2		continue heparin NO warfarin
Day 3	6.0 p.m.	STOP HEPARIN 10 mg warfarin

Day 4	a.m.	Prothrombin time
		5 mg warfarin (if
	p.m.	prothrombin ratio
		2.5 or below)

If the prothrombin time on day 4 is within the therapeutic range or below we continue with 5 mg warfarin as suggested above. If the coagulation time is very prolonged (unusual in our experience) the dose on day 4 can be omitted, the prothrombin time repeated on day 5 and the dose adjusted accordingly. In any event, daily prothrombin times with adjustments of the evening dose are necessary for several days before stability is reached and then weekly estimations are probably sufficient. We have tried other regimens, e.g. starting with 3 consecutive days of 10 mg warfarin daily (said to be more 'physiological') but maintenance dosage takes much longer to achieve this way and we have also had many more dangerously prolonged prothrombin times. It should always be remembered that any desire to withdraw long-term anticoagulant prophylaxis is complicated by an increased risk of embolism after stopping therapy during pregnancy (Hedstrand & Cullhed 1968), particularly during the withdrawal period, presumably due to rebound hyper-coagulability (Poller & Thomson 1964).

Heparin

Heparin is a powerful anticoagulant with a molecular weight that varies between 15 000 and 40 000; as far as is known it does not cross the placenta (Bonnar 1976) and on this basis would appear to be the safest anticoagulant to use during pregnancy (Flessa et al 1974). Unlike warfarin, its effect in vivo can be rapidly reversed by intravenous administration of protamine sulphate which immediately neutralises the effect of heparin, so that emergency surgery can be undertaken and bleeding due to overdosage dealt with promptly. In contrast to warfarin the half-life is a matter of hours, therefore withholding therapy alone will rapidly restore coagulation and haemostasis to normal.

Its main disadvantage is that it has to be given parenterally and, before the introduction of self-administered subcutaneous injections, was only used over the short-term. Its effects on the haemostatic mechanism as a whole are complex but, there are two main alterations in the coagulation factors which can be monitored in vitro. Given prophylactically in small doses subcutaneously, heparin prevents the spontaneous activation of factor X to factor Xa. To treat an established thrombus large doses are given intravenously preferably by continuous infusion starting with 40 000 i.u. daily. Given in large therapeutic doses heparin has a powerful antithrombin effect. It is absorbed onto the clot and prevents further conversion of fibrinogen to fibrin by thrombin. The amount of heparin required to achieve therapeutic levels varies directly with the size of the thrombus, larger doses being required for pulmonary emboli or massive iliofemoral thromboses than for a small deep venous thrombosis, in the calf.

Laboratory monitoring of therapeutic heparin

Several methods of laboratory control of heparin therapy are in current usage. Methods based on prolongation of various in vitro tests of coagulation cascade efficiency notably the partial thromboplastin time (PTT) and the thrombin time (TT) are not very satisfactory. It has been suggested that prolongation of the PTT to 1.5–2 times the normal indicates effective safe anticoagulation. However each individual metabolises heparin differently and the control plasma must be taken from the patient concerned before the heparin infusion is commenced.

It has also been suggested that prolongation of the thrombin time to 2–3 times the normal control indicates a satisfactory level of heparin in the circulation. The same criteria apply to the control plasma as for the partial thrombo-plastin time. We struggled in this laboratory with both these methods for monitoring therapeutic heparin levels for some years but found the methods unsatisfactory. Our results seemed to bear no clinical relationship to what was actually happening in the patient until we decided to try the protamine sulphate neutralisation test.

Protamine sulphate neutralisation test (PSNT). This is an extension of the thrombin clotting time test, in which varying concentrations of protamine sulphate are added to the patient's plasma before the addition of thrombin. When all the heparin in the plasma has been neutralised then the thrombin clotting time will become normal. The amount of heparin in the sample can be calculated from the amount of protamine sulphate needed to neutralise its effect on the thrombin clotting time (Dacie & Lewis 1975).

Therapeutic levels of heparin are considered to lie between 0.5–2.0 i.u./ml. We have found this test for maintaining heparin levels by far the most helpful. It seems to bear a clear relationship to the clinical situation and aids the obstetrician to achieve satisfactory control rather than just confusing the issue. There is one caveat however: it is absolutely essential that any specimen taken for monitoring the heparin level is taken from a site remote from the infusion line and never from the infusion line itself. No amount of 'washing through' will ensure an uncontaminated specimen and the results may cause unwarranted panic!

Subcutaneous heparin

Bonnar (1976a) pioneered the use of self-administered subcutaneous heparin for the treatment and prophylaxis of thrombo-embolism in pregnancy; more than 200 patients have been managed to date using this method. Its efficiency depends on the fact that in doses too small to have a direct effect on thrombin in the circulation, heparin inhibits the activation of factor X to factor Xa, an action almost identical with and potentiated by the naturally occurring anticoagulant anti-thrombin III. Factor X occupies a key linking position in the coagulation cascade (see Fig. 1.2). Small dose prophylactic subcutaneous heparin normally does not require monitoring when given to cover surgery in the presence of normal hepatic and renal function. A standard dose used is 5000 i.u. 8-hourly. During pregnancy, therapy continues for a much longer time and requirements are greater, particularly in the weeks approaching term (Whitfield et al 1983); because of variations in renal function which may occur it has been suggested that frequent monitoring should be undertaken so that dangerous or inadequate anticoagulation can be avoided (Bonnar 1981b). At this hospital heparin activity is estimated at each antenatal visit. The desired levels of heparin do not quantitatively lower the coagulation factors in the plasma and therefore the effect cannot be measured by using the crude biological tests of coagulation activity such as PTT, PT, or TT. The introduction of a more specific assay method based on the ability of heparin to accelerate the neutralisation of factor Xa has allowed these low levels of heparin in the plasma to be measured (Denson & Bonnar 1973). This test is not performed routinely in all laboratories in the United Kingdom, so it is incumbent on any obstetrician caring for a patient on long-term subcutaneous heparin prophylaxis to make arrangements for the plasma to be examined at another laboratory if the test is not available on site, or transfer the patient to the care of a hospital where the laboratory provides that facility. Experience (Bonnar 1981a) suggests that a plasma heparin level of 0.02–0.3 i.u./ml provides adequate prophylaxis against thrombo-embolism without the hazard of bleeding. Our experience would support this observation (see below). Where subcutaneous heparin prophylaxis is used without facilities for monitoring levels, a dose of 7500 i.u. twice daily has been suggested (Bonnar 1981a). We use 10 000 i.u. 12-hourly throughout the antenatal period, only altering the dose by reducing it if levels of more than 0.3 i.u./ml are found (see below). In our experience this only occurs rarely. Postpartum the dose of heparin is reduced to 8000 i.u. b.d.

At the moment ampoules of heparin are only available in aliquots of 5000 i.u. which means that we have to teach women to draw up the appropriate dose into a tuberculin syringe (0.4 ml of 25 000 u/ml is equal to 10 000 i.u.). It would greatly facilitate administration for the women concerned if sterile ampoule packs of 10 000 i.u. were available with needles already attached. Calcium heparin has been shown to have a shorter effect in the circulation than sodium heparin, therefore Bonnar and Ma (1979) recommend the use of sodium heparin 12-hourly for long-term prophylaxis during pregnancy. The platelet count should be monitored as frequently as the heparin level, as there have been reports of heparin-induced thrombocytopenia (Gerwin 1975, Godal 1980, Salzman et al 1980, Cines et al 1980, Rhodes et al 1977, Chong et al 1982).

Mechanism of induction of thrombocytopenia

Thrombocytopenia is a well-recognised complication of heparin therapy with a reported incidence of 1–30% (Malcolm et al 1979, Bell 1976). The pathophysiology is not well understood and remains controversial. Heparin-induced platelet clumping and sequestration, immune mediated platelet destruction and disseminated intravascular coagulation are some of the suggested mechanisms producing thrombocytopenia. A recent prospective study (Chong et al 1982) found that patients could be divided into two distinct groups on clinical grounds — one group had only mild symptomless thrombocytopenia of early onset, the platelet count being above $65 \times 10^9/l$. The mechanisms of the development of this type of thrombocytopenia appeared to be attributable to a direct effect of heparin on the platelet. The second group had severe thrombocytopenia with delayed onset and a high incidence of thrombo-embolic complications with some fatalities. In all of these patients with severe thrombocytopenia of delayed onset a heparin-dependent IgG antibody was found in the serum which activated the platelet prostaglandin pathway and released thromboxane — a powerful aggregating agent. Chong and colleagues (1982) point out that different approaches are needed in the management of these two distinct types of heparin-induced thrombocytopenia. Patients with mild early onset thrombocytopenia need no active treatment but those with severe thrombocytopenia ($<50 \times 10^9/l$) of delayed onset, should be started on oral anticoagulants with or without antiplatelet drugs and the heparin stopped immediately. We have yet to see this complication of heparin therapy, either of the mild or severe delayed type.

Use of anticoagulants during pregnancy

It is established that there is a definite though slight risk of teratogenesis associated with warfarin therapy in the first trimester of pregnancy (Kerber et al 1968, Pettifor and Benson 1975, Abbot et al 1977, Becker et al 1975). It has also been recognised for many years that the use of warfarin during late pregnancy (after 36 weeks gestation) is associated with serious retroplacental and fetal bleeding — an important hazard to the fetus being intracerebral haemorrhage (Villasanta 1965). These hazards can be explained by warfarin crossing the placenta together with the fact that the fetus has low levels of the clotting factors synthesised in the liver, even without the influence of warfarin, because of the liver's functional immaturity. For these reasons Hirsh and colleagues (1970) recommended that, after an initial period of heparisation in the acute attack, heparin should continue to be used for the first trimester followed by warfarin between 13 and 36 weeks, reverting to heparin for the last weeks of pregnancy.

Heparin in low concentrations prevents the activation of factor X, a key substance in both the extrinsic and intrinsic coagulation systems. Given in very small doses prophylactically, replacing warfarin in the first trimester and from 36 weeks to term, heparin will prevent the initiation of thrombosis without actively depressing the synthesis of coagulation factors in the liver (as warfarin does) and therefore the woman so treated is not at risk from haemorrhage during parturition, whether this is achieved by caesarean section or by normal vaginal delivery, nor is the fetus at risk of haemorrhage

41

during delivery. The recommendations of Hirsh and colleagues (1970) have been widely followed (Pridmore et al 1975, Henderson et al 1972, Szekely et al 1973, de Swiet et al 1980, Anon 1975) and a recent survey of obstetric practice in the United Kingdom showed that over 70% of clinicians would still follow them (de Swiet et al 1980). However, as early as 1975, an editorial in the British Medical Journal questioned the use of oral anticoagulants even after the first trimester because of the risk of fetal malformation.

Sherman & Hall (1972) described a case of microcephaly in the newborn infant of a patient who had taken warfarin for the last six months of pregnancy only and this stimulated further correspondence (Carson & Reid 1976, Hall 1976), culminating in a report (Holzgreve et al 1976) in which a further five cases of microcephaly occurring in California were cited. It has been suggested (Shaul & Hall 1977), that the optic atrophy, microcephaly and mental retardation described has been caused by repeated small intercerebral haemorrhages, induced by maternal warfarin therapy.

We have noted bleeding problems in a series of women treated antenatally with warfarin, despite satisfactory therapeutic control (de Swiet et al 1977). Pregnant women may bleed for reasons other than anticoagulant therapy, for example, accidental haemorrhage. Although it is difficult to demonstrate a statistically significant increase in such 'obstetric' causes of bleeding associated with anticoagulant therapy it is our impression that patients are more likely to bleed seriously in such cases if oral anticoagulants are used than if they are not anticoagulated.

Bonnar (1976a) first described the use of long-term self-administered heparin for the prevention and treatment of thrombo-embolic complications during pregnancy. This regimen should obviate the haemorrhagic problem described above in mother and fetus. Therefore, with the exception of patients who are at risk from arterial thrombo-embolism (atrial fibrillation and artificial heart valves, see below), we have now stopped using warfarin during the antenatal period.

Anticoagulant treatment of established thrombo-embolism during pregnancy

Initial anticoagulant treatment of a deep venous thrombosis or pulmonary embolism always involves parenteral administration of heparin, whether in the antenatal period or not because heparin exerts its powerful anticoagulant effect immediately. The heparin is delivered by continuous intravenous infusion to achieve a level of 0.5–1.5 (or 1–2) i.u./ml. The initial dose is 40 000 i.u. over the first 24 hours, and is monitored by the protamine sulphate neutralisation test (see above), the dose adjusted accordingly to obtain the desired concentration. More heparin will be required in those cases with large thromboses (see above). After an arbitrary period of 5 days (more in more severe cases, less in trivial cases) the therapy is, in the antenatal period, changed to self-administered subcutaneous heparin 10 000 i.u. b.d. monitored by factor Xa Assay (Denson & Bonnar 1973). Provided that there is detectable activity using the factor Xa assay the dose of heparin should not be altered to increase the activity. There is no evidence that keeping the level between 0.1–0.3 units per ml is in any way more effective than a detectable level in vitro below 0.1 i.u. per ml. If the heparin assay detects levels of 0.3 i.u. per ml or above it is necessary to lower the dose because these levels are approaching the therapeutic range and can be associated with excessive bleeding at delivery (Bonnar 1975) especially if there is surgical intervention. Subcutaneous small-dose heparin levels are stable in patients outside pregnancy with normal renal function and usually do not have to be monitored. During pregnancy, however, therapy may have to be continued for unusually long periods — months, rather than days or weeks — and the changing plasma volume combined with possible impairment of renal function make frequent factor Xa assay advisable if dangerously high levels are to be avoided. Measurements of heparin levels are made at each antenatal visit, which means a weekly estimation in the last month.

Impaired renal excretion will result in unexpectedly high levels of heparin and, in our experience, may precede failure to control hypertension in the course of pre-eclampsia and other conditions, and warn the obstetrician of imminent danger to the patient.

Anticoagulation during labour

Because of the high incidence of thrombo-embolism in the days following labour and delivery and the increased risk following operative delivery, subcutaneous heparin is continued throughout labour and delivery whether it be normal vaginal, instrumental or by caesarean section. The heparin assay is checked in the week preceding delivery (see above). A small controlled trial of prophylactic subcutaneous heparin therapy (Howell et al 1983) showed no excess of antenatal or postnatal bleeding associated with small-dose heparin. Average estimated postpartum blood loss in the treated group was 188 ml with a mean of 215 ml in the controls. These estimations are notoriously inaccurate, but there was no obvious difference between the two groups. Epidural anaesthesia is contraindicated, however, in all patients receiving anticoagulants because of the risk of epidural haematoma formation which could have disastrous permanent effects (Crawford 1980). This hazard is probably remote in association with subcutaneous small-dose heparin therapy, but the risk should not be taken.

Postpartum therapy

Therapy is continued for an arbitrary period of 6 weeks postpartum at which time the extra risk of thrombo-embolism associated with pregnancy is considered to have passed. This time was extended from 3 weeks to 6 weeks after one of our patients developed a recurrent deep vein thrombosis in the 5th week. The majority of obstetricians in the United Kingdom treat patients continuously for 6 weeks in the puerperium (de Swiet et al 1980). The risk of bleeding from secondary postpartum haemorrhage continues for at least 10 days postpartum. Severe secondary postpartum haemorrhage was observed in several women on warfarin in our initial study (de Swiet et al 1977). We therefore continued to use heparin in this period. Most women who require treatment in the puerperium for thrombo-embolism sustained in the recent pregnancy or for prophylaxis (see below) will be remaining in hospital for 8–10 days postdelivery anyway. After a week to 10 days we change those women who wish to stop subcutaneous injections to warfarin even if they are breast feeding. It has been shown (Orme et al 1977) that there is no detectable secretion of warfarin in the breast milk, and that infants who are breast fed while their mothers are taking warfarin are not at any increased risk of abnormal bleeding unlike those breast-fed infants whose mothers were taking phenindione (Eckstein & Jack 1970). The disadvantage of switching to warfarin is that the mother has to make quite frequent hospital visits so that citrated blood can be taken for estimation of the prothrombin time and the warfarin dose adjusted accordingly. No monitoring of heparin therapy is required in the puerperium, but there is the disadvantage of continuing with twice daily subcutaneous injections for 6 weeks postpartum.

The prophylaxis of thrombo-embolism

There are two groups of patients in whom prophylaxis might be considered:

1. Those who are at high risk because of age, parity, obesity or operative delivery (DHSS 1982).
2. Those who have had a thrombo-embolism in the past (Badaracco & Vessey 1974).

In regard to the first group it is generally believed, though not proven, that the risk of thrombo-embolism is greatest in the postnatal period and that any prophylaxis need only be used to cover labour and the puerperium. The Confidential Enquiries into Maternal Mortality (DHSS 1982) shows clearly that the risks of thrombo-embolism increase with high parity and increasing age. These factors are independent of each other. It would seem reasonable to use some form of prophylaxis for all patients over 30 years having a caesarean section and also in women over 35 years even if they have a normal vaginal delivery. However, subcutaneous heparin used widely in other forms of surgery is not necessarily the best choice. Its use would preclude epidural anaesthesia (see above) and it probably would have to be given before the onset of labour to be effective.

Intravenous dextran administered during labour or caesarean section may be a better choice for prophylaxis of thrombo-embolism — dextran affects platelet function and reduces their adhesiveness and aggregation. Thrombi formed in its presence are more easily lysed; the reasons for this being so are not understood. However, it also interferes with compatibility tests required for blood transfusion therefore uncontaminated blood should be taken before the dextran infusion is started and used for cross-matching purposes should blood transfusion be required. We know of no systematic evaluation of the efficacy and risks of dextran infusions to prevent thrombo-embolism during pregnancy, although there have been differing reports of its efficacy in other situations (Morris & Mitchell 1978). Two large studies have shown that dextran infusions are effective in reducing the incidence of fatal postoperative pulmonary embolism. (Kline et al 1975, Gruber et al 1980). Dextran should be avoided in any obstetric patient with cardiac or renal impairment or with a history of allergic reactions, as rarely, dextran can cause anaphylaxis. A recent survey involving over 200 clinics in Sweden showed that approximately 12% of clinicians do not use dextran 70 for prophylaxis because of the risk of serious anaphylactic reactions (Bergquist 1980). Also it has been suggested that the bleeding problems using dextran 40 can approach the frequency of those encountered with oral anticoagulants (Harris et al 1972). Nevertheless, Bonnar (1979) suggests that dextran 70 can be used in patients having epidural anaethesia. Dextran should be avoided in any patient receiving heparin as the two agents have a synergistic effect which thus increases the hazard of serious haemorrhage (Bonnar 1979).

The second group of patients, those having had thrombo-embolism in the past, are thought to be at risk throughout pregnancy. Badaracco & Vessey (1974) estimated that there was about a 12% risk of developing a pulmonary embolism or deep vein thrombosis during pregnancy in patients who had had previous thrombo-embolism in the past. The risk was the same whether the original thrombosis was associated with the contraceptive pill or not, but the study was retrospective.

A survey of the use of anticoagulant by obstetricians in the United Kingdom (de Swiet et al 1980) showed that most (88%) would use prophylactic anticoagulants for a woman who had had a previous thrombo-embolism during pregnancy or whilst taking the contraceptive pill (73%). However, only 50% of the obstetricians co-operating in the survey would use prophylaxis if the woman had had a thrombo-embolism 10 years previously when she was neither pregnant nor taking 'the pill'! The majority of obstetricians would still use the modified Hirsh regimen of warfarin from 14 to 36 weeks gestation and then switch to subcutaneous heparin. For reasons cited above we do not advocate the use of warfarin in the antenatal period except in association with artificial heart valves, mitral valve disease and fibrillation (see below).

Does self-administered subcutaneous heparin prophylaxis throughout pregnancy have any disadvantages and does it really reduce the incidence of thrombo-embolism? Only a large study with multi-centre co-operation could answer these questions satisfactorily because the numbers at risk in any one centre are small. In an attempt to stimulate such an investigation we have just completed a small prospective controlled trial of antenatal prophylaxis against thrombo-embolism (Howell et al 1983). Twenty randomly chosen patients with a documented history of previous thrombo-embolism received heparin 10 000 i.u. subcutaneously twice daily throughout pregnancy; another similarly chosen 20 patients were allotted to the no-treatment group, to evaluate possible side effects knowing that a much larger study would be required to prove the efficacy of such treatment in pregnancy.

Although heparin does not cross the placenta it has been suggested that there is a high morbidity in the babies of mothers so treated (Hall et al 1980). This morbidity and mortality arises from abortion and prematurity. The most obvious maternal complication is bruising at the injection site. This can be reduced by good injection technique but never eliminated. Most mothers tolerate this degree of bruising, inconvenient and sometimes painful as it is. A very serious complication of prolonged heparin administration, which is not generally recognised, is a form of bone demineralisation described as osteopenia (Avioli 1975). The cause of this osteopenia is unknown although it has been attributed to a deficiency of 1,2-dihydrotachysterol (Aarskog et al 1980). It has also been reported (Rhodes et al 1977, Cines et al 1980) that heparin may cause thrombocytopenia sufficient to result in bleeding, or be associated with serious thrombotic complications (Chong et al 1982). The disadvantages of heparin therapy seem to be associated with the antenatal period — abortion and prematurity for the fetus and thrombocytopenia, osteopenia and avoidance of epidural anaesthesia for the mother. Therefore, both the control patients and treated patients in our trial were given subcutaneous heparin during the puerperium. All patients received 8000 i.u. heparin 12-hourly for 6 weeks from the first postnatal day. There appeared to be no increased risk of antenatal or postnatal bleeding associated with heparin but 1 patient in the control group developed a deep venous thrombosis antenatally, for which she was treated promptly. One patient in the treatment group developed severe debilitating osteopenia resulting in a collapsed vertebrae diagnosed in the puerperium. Preliminary studies suggest that some degree of bone demineralisation occurs in all patients on long-term heparin (de Swiet et al 1983). Thrombocytopenia was not a problem in our patients as previously reported (Cines et al 1980). The avoidance of epidural anaesthesia may have contributed to both maternal and fetal morbidity in the treatment group. The increased risk of fetal wastage associated with antenatal heparin prophylaxis due to prematurity and abortion (Hall et al 1980) was not substantiated by our small trial, but admissions to the special care baby unit were greater in the treatment group (25%) as compared to the control group (10%). This study, which to our knowledge is the only randomised controlled trial of anticoagulant prophylaxis during pregnancy, does suggest that subcutaneous heparin is not without risks to both the mother and fetus, apart from the discomfort of twice daily subcutaneous injections over a relatively long period. The place of heparin prophylaxis therefore remains uncertain, particularly when we are trying to compare maternal benefits (i.e. reducing the incidence of pulmonary embolism) with fetal risks. A larger series would allow more precise quantification of both fetal and maternal risks together with possible maternal benefit. An alternative approach would be to accept that the period of maximum risk for recurrent thrombo-embolism during any pregnancy is in the puerperium and to take measures to cover this period only (Letsky & de Swiet 1984). During labour and delivery intravenous dextran could be administered (Bergquist et al 1980), which would allow the use of epidural anaesthesia. After delivery the mother could be treated with subcutaneous heparin and switched to warfarin if she so desires after 1 week to complete a 6-week prophylaxis period in the puerperium.

It is now our policy to follow the above regimen. There is close antenatal supervision of all patients with a history of previous thrombo-embolism. They are encouraged to attend the hospital at the slightest suspicion of a developing DVT, cough or chest-pain, and are seen by the physician regularly at routine antenatal visits, as well as by the obstetrician. Of course any diagnosed thrombo-embolism is treated promptly following the regimen indicated previously. Dextran is given to cover labour and delivery and then the patient is switched to subcutaneous heparin alone or progressing to warfarin for 6 weeks during puerperium. Nevertheless this remains an uneasy compromise for patients could still die in the antenatal period from pulmonary embolism.

Prophylaxis of thrombo-embolism during pregnancy for women with artificial heart valves

While small-dose subcutaneous heparin, complications aside, seems to be an effective constituent of management regimes for prophylaxis and treatment of venous thrombo-embolism this is not the case for patients at risk from arterial thrombo-embolism (Duncan 1978, Oakley 1983). These constitute patients with artificial heart valves, those with mitral valve disease and/or artrial fibrillation. The pathogenesis of thrombo-embolism is presumably different in these cases where there is a foreign body in the circulation or markedly abnormal patterns of blood flow. Naturally occurring fibrinolytic mechanisms are less active in the wall of arteries than in veins, women who require valve replacements should ideally have homograft or xenograft tissue valves. However, there is still concern about the longevity of such valves (Cohn et al 1981, Kirklin 1981) and it is likely that women will continue to receive artificial heart valves even if they plan to have children. The efficacy of subcutaneous heparin prophylaxis has not been substantiated in patients with artificial heart valves. Fatal thrombo-embolism has been reported in pregnancy where such treatment was used for a mother with a mitral prosthesis (Bennett & Oakley 1968). The addition of antiplatelet agents such as dipyridamole may help in individual cases (Biale et al 1977) but the general efficacy of such measures has not been proven. We therefore continue to use warfarin in these patients acknowledging that such treatment must remain an uneasy compromise. The risk of teratogenecity in the first trimester, though present, is small.

We have recently reviewed the babies of 22 women who took warfarin in pregnancy and compared them with matched controls. Two women took warfarin throughout pregnancy. 16 took warfarin in the second and third trimesters and the remainder took warfarin in the third trimester only. There was no difference in developmental scores between the treated babies and their controls and no clinical or radiological evidence of chondrodysplasia in the treated babies. In addition a further 6 children exposed to warfarin in pregnancy were reported as normal by their general practitioners. These 28 children were drawn from a total population of 46 pregnancies treated with warfarin amongst which there was a high perinatal mortality, with 2 stillbirths and 2 neonatal deaths. Another recent study (Chen et al 1982) suggests that the fetal risks of warfarin therapy are not so great as had been previously suspected.

The first cases of chondrodysplasia punctata were all described in women with artifical heart valves who entered pregnancy already on warfarin maintenance therapy (Kerber et al 1968, Pettifor & Benson 1978, Abbot et al 1977, Becker et al 1975). It has been suggested that patients with artificial heart valves should use heparin in the first trimester (Oakley & Doherty 1976) but this is not practical. Small-dose subcutaneous heparin has been shown to be ineffective in this situation, therefore high-dose intravenous heparin should be used — patients cannot say exactly when they will conceive and it is difficult to envisage the exact circumstances in which they could become pregnant with a constant intravenous heparin infusion running! We advise patients to continue with warfarin, accepting the risk to the fetus and the small risk of bleeding until about 36 weeks gestation when the risk of fetal intracerebral and retroplancental haemorrhage seems overwhelming. Monitoring of warfarin has to be undertaken more frequently than when nonpregnant because of changing plasma volume and levels of coagulation factors. At 36 weeks, assuming that the cervix is favourable for induction, the woman is admitted to hospital and warfarin therapy stopped. The woman is started on a continuous intravenous infusion of heparin to produce a level of 0.8–1.0 i.u./ml using the PSNT*. This treatment is continued for 10 days. By this time the effects of warfarin will have worn off and the patient can be delivered either vaginally or by caesarean section under heparin cover, but at a reduced dose to achieve a level of 0.4–0.6 i.u./ml. Warfarin is recommenced 5–7 days postpartum. ˙

Neutralising anticoagulant therapy

In rare situations the effect of heparin or warfarin may have to be reversed because of bleeding or the need to undertake urgent surgery, most commonly caesarean section, at a time when the patient is in a hypocoagulable state.

Heparin has a short half-life administered conventionally (see aerosol administration below) and stopping the drug or decreasing the dosage is usually sufficient. Occasionally protamine sulphate may have to be given to neutralise the effect. For every 100 i.u. heparin in the circulation 1 mg of protamine sulphate is given.

A simple formula for calculating the neutralising dose of protamine sulphate is as follows (see Ingram et al 1982):

$$\text{Protamine sulphate required (mg) to neutralise heparin} = \text{plasma heparin concentration i.u./ml} \times \text{plasma volume} \times 0.01$$

Plasma volume during pregnancy may be taken as 50 ml per kilogram body weight. For example a woman of 65 kilogram with a plasma heparin concentration of 0.8 i.u./ml would require

$$0.8 \times (65 \times 50) \times .01 = 26 \text{ mg protamine sulphate}$$

Remember to allow for the rapid clearance of heparin from the blood and also that in excess protamine sulphate can act as an anticoagulant itself. Unless there is a dire emergency, either copious bleeding or the necessity to perform urgent caesarean section, it is better to wait until the heparin is metabolised rather than to actively intervene.

---

*See p. 38.

The effect of warfarin can only be reversed immediately by the administration of 1–2 units of fresh frozen plasma. Vitamin K administered orally or intravenously will reverse the effect of warfarin in 24 hours. Where a firm decision has been taken not to reintroduce anticoagulants, a dose of 25–50 mg will render the patient resistant to further anticoagulant treatment for 2 weeks or more. Where continued therapy is desirable in the face of haemorrhage, 15 mg vitamin K should be given to reduce the drug effect. If routine prothrombin times shows excessive prolongation without bleeding a dose of 5 mg can be given (Bonnar 1979).

Antithrombin III

Antithrombin III (AtIII) is an important naturally occurring physiological inhibitor of blood clotting. Despite progress in the field, the factors that promote coagulation are far better defined than those that inhibit it. AtIII is the main physiological inhibitor of thrombin and factor Xa and possibly the main inhibitor of factors IXa, XIa and XIIa (Abildgaard 1981). An inherited deficiency of AtIII is one of the very few conditions in which a familial tendency to thrombosis has been described (see below).

Heparin (see above) is the oldest anticoagulant drug and has been in clinical use for over 40 years (Barrowcliffe et al 1978). It remains the most potent anticoagulant drug available. Heparin markedly accelerates the rate at which AtIII reacts to thrombin and factor Xa. The interaction between heparin and AtIII is of considerable clinical importance in the treatment and prophylaxis of thrombo-embolism (Barrowcliffe & Thomas 1981).

Six different types of antithrombin have been described but only the first three have been shown to play any significant role in haemostasis (Lane & Biggs 1977). The activity in plasma which causes progressive destruction of thrombin was originally termed 'antithrombin III'. It is now recognised that at least three proteins contribute towards this activity — two general proteinase inhibitors, α_1 antitrypsin and α_2 macroglobulin and α_2 globulin with more specific antithrombin activity, now known as antithrombin III. Addition of a specific antibody to AtIII removes all the heparin cofactor activity from plasma and the evidence is overwhelming that these factors are identical. AtIII, therefore, is not only the major thrombin inhibitor in plasma but is also the plasma protein through which heparin exerts its effect (Barrowcliffe & Thomas 1981). As

51

AtIII is synthesised in the liver, its activity is low in cirrhosis and other chronic deseases of the liver as well as in protein-losing renal disease, DIC and hypercoagulable states.

The commonest cause of a small reduction in plasma AtIII is use of oral contraceptives (Fagerhol & Abildgaard 1970, Howie et al 1970, Von Kaulla & Von Kaulla 1970). In the past 20 years it has become obvious that there is a causal relationship between oral contraceptive steroids and venous thrombo-embolism, though this role in thrombopathogenesis has not been fully evaluated. It is obvious that the oestrogen content is important and since the introduction of low-dose oestrogen pills the associated incidence of venous thrombo-embolism has fallen dramatically (Bottiger et al 1980). A significant fall in AtIII has been found in women taking oestroprogestagens, regardless of the oestrogen content, but not in association with progestagen-only pills (Conard et al 1980).

The depression of AtIII activity may not be the only factor involved in the association of oestrogen-containing oral contraceptives with thrombo-embolism; oestrogen itself may cause endothelial injury. An increase in plasma-antiplasmin has also been demonstrated (Howie et al 1970).

In a retrospective analysis of the plasma of 50 contraceptive pill-taking women, 6–12 months after an episode of thrombo-embolus, none had demonstrable AtIII deficiency but over 30% had defective fibrinolytic activity (Bergquist et al 1982). In a prospective study of antithrombin III (XaI) activity associated with low-dose oestrogen oral contraceptives, there was a significant reduction in XaI activity after 1 month of oestrogen consumption but no significant difference between those women taking 30 μg and 50 μg in terms of AtIII levels (Bergquist et al 1983). Accumulating evidence suggests that suppression of AtIII is only one of many contributory interacting risk factors associated with venous thrombo-embolism and oestrogen-containing oral contraceptives. During uncomplicated pregnancy a slight lowering of antifactor Xa and AtIII have been found towards term (Biland & Duckett 1973, Bonnar 1976b) though another more recent study showed no change in AtIII levels during pregnancy itself (Hellgren & Blomback 1981), but some lowering during delivery and then an increase 1 week postpartum. The authors suggest that AtIII synthesis must be increased during pregnancy to maintain normal mean levels in the face of increasing plasma volume. The principle of laboratory measurement of biological activity of AtIII depends on its ability to neutralise thrombin or factor Xa. Fixed amounts of thrombin or factor Xa are added to dilutions of the test plasma and the residual enzyme activity measured immunologically using monospecific antisera but this will give no indication of its biological activity. In clinical laboratories the advent of chromogenic substances for the measurement of thrombin and factor Xa has had a major impact on the measurement of AtIII activity, but these recently available commercial kits vary in sensitivity and may not measure all the bioactivity. For the time being it would seem sensible not to rely solely on values of AtIII estimated by only one of the main types of assay (Barrowcliffe & Thomas 1981).

Inherited antithrombin III deficiency

The first report of inherited antithrombin III deficiency in a family with a remarkably high incidence of venous thrombo-embolic problems came from Norway (Egeberg 1965). Thrombo-embolism occurred most often in association with inflammation, trauma, surgical operations and pregnancy. Family members with a history of thrombosis, and some of their children, were found to have abnormally low levels of AtIII with an average value of 50% of normal, measured both by a biological and an immunological method. Numerous other families with this autosomal dominant inherited defect have now been reported and an increased associated incidence of thrombo-embolism has been repeatedly confirmed in the last decade (Johansson et al 1978, Nagy et al 1979, Abildgaard 1981, Anon 1983, Ambruso et al 1980). The risk of thrombo-embolism in women with congenital AtIII deficiency is further increased during pregnancy (Brandt & Stendjberg 1975, Egeberg 1965, Johansson et al 1978). Pregnancy per se, obstetric complications and delivery may lower AtIII in women without an inherited deficiency (Bonnar 1977, Buller et al 1980, Hellgren & Blomback 1981). Heparin has been used successfully for prophylaxis and treatment of women in pregnancy with normal AtIII levels (see above) (Hellgren and Nygards 1981, Spearing et al 1978, Bonnar 1979) and prophylaxis of thrombo-embolism with heparin and other agents has also been reported in women with congenital or acquired AtIII deficiency (Blomback & Kockum 1974, Brandt & Stendjberg 1979, Johanssen et al 1978).

For reasons given above warfarin should be avoided during pregnancy and the early puerperium. Patients with low AtIII activity undergoing surgical operation also respond to short-term low-dose subcutaneous heparin prophylaxis. However, in patients given heparin intravenously over a long period with initial acquired low

AtIII activity, the therapy may be ineffectual and result in even lower levels of AtIII activity.

Small-dose subcutaneous heparin prophylaxis has proved to be ineffective in preventing thrombo-embolism in pregnant women with congenital AtIII deficiency (Blomback & Kockum 1974, Brandt & Stendjberg 1979). Purified preparations of AtIII prepared from plasma are now available and have been administered during pregnancy to women with acquired and congenital AtIII deficiency (Buller et al 1980, Hellgen et al 1981). The half-life of AtIII is around three days and is shortened in the presence of heparin. The incidence of thrombo-embolic complications during pregnancy in women with congenital AtIII deficiency has been estimated retrospectively to be approximately 70% (Hellgren et al 1981).

One regimen for successful prophylaxis of thrombo-embolism in women with AtIII during pregnancy has been suggested following a prospective study (Hellgren et al 1981). The woman should receive subcutaneous heparin or intravenous heparin to achieve levels within the therapeutic range, i.e. significant prolongation of the PTT or protamine sulphate neutralisation giving heparin levels around 0.8–1.0 i.u./ml. At delivery or abortion the antithrombin level should be brought to normal by infusion of AtIII concentrate and the heparin reduced or withdrawn to avoid bleeding. In the antenatal period it was found that during administration of heparin the AtIII level dropped even further to around 25% of normal. The heparin requirements were increased to reach the desired prolongation of the PTT compared with the requirement in the presence of normal AtIII levels but the desired effect could always be obtained. No adverse reactions (allergic pyrogenic) were noted during administration of pure AtIII concentrate but one woman developed non-A non-B hepatitis following administration of the concentrate plus fresh frozen plasma. Another woman who received the same batch of concentrated AtIII but no fresh frozen plasma had no adverse effect (Hellgren et al 1981).

The incidence of inherited AtIII deficiency is unknown and probably varies in different populations but it is not common. Abildgaard (1981) suggested an incidence of 1 in 5000 arising from the finding of 5 women with congenital deficiency in 25 000 pill users in Scandinavia. Therefore it would be unrealistic to screen every woman at booking for this rare defect. However, it is sensible to check the AtIII in any woman who has a previous history of thrombo-embolism (a rare event in any woman in the reproductive years) because, if she has low AtIII, routine heparin prophylaxis is ineffective during pregnancy. Larger doses of subcutaneous or intravenous heparin to produce prolongation of clotting times are recommended together with AtIII concentrates at delivery.

Screening for women at risk for thrombo-embolism during pregnancy

There is no point in mass screening for women at risk with the methods available to date because no single screening technique for detecting an increased risk of thrombo-embolism associated with pregnancy has been found. Discriminant analysis has shown fibrinopeptide A, fibrinogen, factor VIIIC, antithrombin III and plasmin activator to be valuable pointers (Hellgren 1981). In addition α_2 antiplasmin and urokinase inhibitors may be of use in individual patients but improved methods for studying blood coagulation and fibrinolysis are necessary in order to find useful predictors of thrombo-embolism during pregnancy.

Other ways of giving heparin

Heparin as aerosol

One of the main disadvantages of long-term heparic prophylaxis is the fact that it has to be given intravenously or subcutaneously. It has a very short half-life and requires repeated injections daily (or continuous infusion). In 1973 the first report of the use of heparin in the form of an aerosol appeared: it described long-term prophylaxis in patients with cardiovascular disease and thrombotic tendencies (Molino & Belluardo 1973). It was shown subsequently that a single dose of heparin administered as an aerosol resulted in a prolonged state of hypocoagulability in dogs, mice and 3 human volunteers (Jacques et al 1976). Following this preliminary report Hellgren and colleagues investigated the effect of heparin aerosol in 16 healthy human volunteers (Hellgren et al 1981), showing that a prolonged anticoagulation effect can be achieved by inhalation of heparin; in some cases the effect lasted for 2–3 weeks. There were no adverse effects such as discomfort, changes in respiratory or cirulatory parameters or allergic reactions. Platelet counts were normal throughout the study. The variable response could be explained by variations in breathing techniques and lung function. A similar variation in response to inhalation of heparin was found in another study (Wrigth & Jacques 1979). The prolonged effect may be brought about by slow release of heparin from macrophages (Jacques & Mahadoo 1978). The difficulty in predicting individual response and the problem of neutralising the prolonged effect of heparin administered in this way should bleeding complications occur, appears to preclude its use in obstetric practice, but the aerosol method of heparin administration certainly deserves further investigation.

Ultra low-dose heparin

The mode of action of low-dose heparin in preventing venous thrombo-embolism may be more complex than was thought. A recent randomised double blind trial of very low-dose intravenous heparin (1 i.u./kg/h) over 3–5 days postoperatively compared favourably with other trials of subcutaneous heparin in preventing thrombo-embolism (Kakkar et al 1978). As would be expected with such a low dose of intravenous heparin there was no increased bleeding in the treated as compared with the control group, but to establish a reduction in postoperative wound haematomata with doses of around 1700 i.u. heparin daily as opposed to 15–20 000 i.u. in 24 hours on conventional subcutaneous prophylaxis requires a much larger clinical trial (Kakkar et al 1978, Negus et al 1980). The response to such small doses of heparin intravenously suggest that it acts as a trigger releasing material which contributes overall to the antithrombotic effect. Support for the concept of release of endogenous material triggered by small doses of heparin is found in two other studies using semisynthetic heparin analogues with very little anticoagulant activity in vitro (Kakkar et al 1978, Hugo et al 1981). Further clinical trials will be necessary before the role of 'ultra low-dose' intravenous heparin, high-dose subcutaneous heparin and heparin analogues can be properly assessed (Barrowcliffe & Thomas 1981).

REFERENCES

Aaro L A, Juergens J L 1971 Thrombophlebitis associated with pregnancy. American Journal of Obstetrics and Gynecology 109: 1128–1136
Aarskog D, Aksnes L, Lehmann V 1980 Low 1,25-dihydroxy vitamin D in heparin-induced osteopenia. Lancet ii: 650–651

Abbott A, Sibert J R, Weaver J B 1977 Chondrodysplasia punctata and maternal warfarin therapy. British Medical Journal i: 1639–1640

Abildgaard U 1981 Antithrombin and related inhibitors of coagulation. In: Pollar C (ed) Recent advances in blood coagulation. Churchill Livingstone, Edinburgh, vol 3, p 151–175

Albrechtsson U, Olsson C-G 1976 Thrombotic side-effects of lower limb phlebography. Lancet i: 728–724

Ambruso D R, Jacobson L J, Hathaway W E 1980 Inherited antithrombin III deficiency and cerebral thrombosis in a child. Pediatrics 65: 125–131

Anon 1975 Venous thrombo-embolism and anticoagulants in pregnancy. British Medical Journal ii: 421–422

Anon 1983 Familial antithrombin III deficiency. Lancet i: 1021–1022

Avioli L V 1975 Heparin-induced osteopenia: an appraisal. Advances in Experimental Medical Biology 52: 375–387

Badaracco M A, Vessey M 1974 Recurrence of venous thrombo-embolic disease and use of oral contraceptives. British Medical Journal i: 215–217

Barrowcliffe T W, Johnson E A, Thomas D 1978 Antithrombin III and heparin. British Medical Bulletin 34: 143–150

Barrowcliffe T W, Thomas D P 1981 Antithrombin III and heparin. In: Bloom A L, Thomas D P (eds) Haemostasis and Thrombosis, Churchill Livingstone, Edinburgh, p 712–724

Becker M H, Genieser N B, Fengold M 1975 Chondrodysplasia punctata: is maternal warfarin therapy a factor. American Journal of Diseases of Children 129: 356–359

Bell W R 1976 Thrombocytopenia occurring during heparin therapy. New England Journal of Medicine 295: 276–277

Bennett G G, Oakley C M 1968 Pregnancy in a patient with mitral valve prosthesis. Lancet i: 616–619

Bergquist A, Bergquist D, Hallbrook T 1979 Acute deep vein thrombosis (DVT) after caesarean section. Acta obstetrica et gynecologica scandinavica 58: 473–476

Bergquist A, Bergquist D, Hedner U 1982 Oral contraceptives and venous thrombo-embolism. British Journal of Obstetrics and Gynaecology 89: 381–386

Bergquist A, Bergquist D, Tangen O 1983 The influence of oral contraceptives on XaI (antithrombin III) activity. A prospective study. British Journal of Obstetrics and Gynaecology (in press)

Bergquist D 1980 Prevention of postoperative thrombosis in Sweden. Results of a survey. World Journal of Surgery 4: 489–495

Biale Y, Lewenthal H, Gueron M, Ben-adereth N 1977 Caesarean section in patients with mitral valve prostheses. Lancet i: 907

Biland L, Duckert F 1973 Coagulation factors of the newborn and his mother. Thrombosis et diathesis haemorrhagica 29: 644–651

Blömback M, Kockum G 1974 Preliminary report on some cases of hereditary antithrombin III deficiency in Sweden. Mexican Journal of Haematology 12: 273–276

Bonnar J 1975 Thrombo-embolism in obstetric and gynaecological patients. In: Nicolaides A W (ed) Thrombo-embolism aetiology. Advances in prevention and management. Medical and Technical Publishing Co Ltd, Lancaster, p 311–341

Bonnar J 1976a Long-term self-administered herapin therapy for prevention and treatment of thrombo-embolic complications in pregnancy. In: Kakkar V V, Thomas D P (eds) Heparin chemistry and clinical usage. Academic Press, London, p 247–260

Bonnar J 1976b Coagulation disorders. Journal of Clinical Pathology 29 (supplement 10) 35–41

Bonnar J 1977 Acute and chronic coagulation problems in pregnancy. In:

L Poller (ed) Recent advances in blood coagulation, Churchill Livingstone, Edinburgh, p 363–378

Bonnar J 1979 Venous thrombo-embolism and pregnancy. In: Stallworthy J, Bourne G (eds) Recent advances in obstetrics and gynaecology, Churchill Livingstone, Edinburgh, p 173–192

Bonnar J 1981a Venous thrombo-embolism and pregnancy. Clinics in obstetrics and gynaecology 8: no. 2 W B Saunders Co. Ltd, p 455–473

Bonnar J 1981b Haemostasis and coagulation disorders in pregnancy. In: Bloom A L, Thomas D P (eds) Haemostasis and thrombosis, Churchill Livingstone, Edinburgh, p 454–471

Bonnar J, Ma P (1979) Prevention of venous thrombo-embolism in pregnancy with subcutaneous sodium and calcium heparin. Proceedings of the IXth World Congress of Gynecology and Obstetrics, Tokyo

Bonnar J, McNicol G P, Douglas A S (1970) Coagulation and fibrinolytic mechanisms during and after normal childbirth. British Medical Journal ii: 200–203

Bottiger L E, Boman G, Eklun D G, Westerhold B 1980 Oral contraception and thrombo-embolic disease: effects of lowering oestrogen content. Lancet i: 1097–1101

Brandt P, Stendjberg S 1979 Subcutaneous heparin for thrombosis in pregnant women with hereditary antithrombin deficiency. Lancet i: 100–101

Browse N 1978 Diagnosis of deep vein thrombosis. British Medical Bulletin 34: 163–167

Büller H R, Weenik A H, Treffers O E, Kahle L H, Otten H A, Tengate J W 1980 Severe antithrombin III deficiency in a patient with pre-eclampsia. Scandinavian Journal of Haematology 25: 81–86

Carson M, Reid M 1976 Warfarin and fetal abnormality. Lancet i: 1127

Chen W W C, Shan C S, Lee P K, Wang R Y C, Wong V C W 1982 Pregnancy in patients with prosthetic heart valves, An experience with 45 pregnancies. The Quarterly Journal of Medicine 51: 358–365

Chong B H, Pitney W R, Castaldi P A 1982 Heparin-induced thrombocytopenia. Association of thrombotic complications with heparin-dependent IgG antibody that induces thromboxane synthesis and platelet aggregation. Lancet ii: 1246–1249

Cines D B, Kaywin P, Bina M, Tomaski A, Schreiber A D 1980 Heparin associated thrombocytopenia. New England Journal of Medicine 303: 788–795

Cohn L H, Mudge G H, Pratter F, Collins J J 1981 Five to eight-year follow-up of patients undergoing porcine heart-valve replacement. New England Journal of Medicine 304: 258–262

Conard J, Cazenave B, Samama M, Horellou M H, Zorn J R. Neau C 1980 AtIII content and antithrombin activity in oestrogen-progestogen and progestogen-only treated women. Thrombosis Research 18: 675–681

Crawford J S 1978, In: Principles and practice of obstetric anaesthesia, 4th edn. Blackwell Scientific Publications, Oxford, p 182–183

Dacie J V D, Lewis S M 1976 Plasma heparin assay. In: Practical haematology, Churchill Livingstone, Edinburgh, p 413–414

Denson K W E, Bonnar J 1973 The measurement of heparin — a method based on the potentiation of antifactor Xa. Thrombosis et diathesis haemorrhagica 30: 471–479

Department of Health and Social Security 1982 Report on Confidential Enquiries into Maternal deaths in England and Wales 1976–78, HMSO, London

Duncan S L B 1978 Long-term self-administered subcutaneous heparin in pregnancy. British Medical Journal ii: 125

Eckstein H, Jack B 1970 Breast feeding and anticoagulant therapy. Lancet i: 672–673

Egeberg O 1965 Inherited antithrombin deficiency causing thrombophilia. Thrombosis et diathesis haemorrhagica 13: 516–530

Exis R, Graeme B C 1974 Congenital athyroidism in the newborn infant from intrauterine radioactive action. Biology of the Neonate 24: 289–291

Fagerhol M K, Abildgaard U 1970 Immunological studies on human antithrombin III influence of age, sex and use or oral contraceptives on serum concentration. Scandinavian Journal of Haematology 7: 10–17

Flanigan D P Goodreau J J, Burnham S J, Gergan J J and Yao J S T 1978 Vascular laboratory diagnosis of clinically suspected acute deep vein thrombosis. Lancet ii: 331–334

Gerwin A S 1975 Complications of heparin therapy. Surgery, Gynecology and Obstetrics 140: 789–796

Godal H C 1980 Thrombocytopenia and heparin. Thrombosis and Haemostasis 43: 222–224

Gruber U F et al 1980 Incidences of fatal postoperative pulmonary embolism after prophylaxis with dextran 70 and low-dose heparin: an international multicentre study. British Medical Journal 280: 69–72

Hall J G 1976 Warfarin and fetal abnormality. Lancet i: 1127

Hall J G, Pauli R M, Wilson K M 1980 Maternal and fetal sequelae of anticoagulation during pregnancy. American Journal of Medicine 68: 122–140

Harris W H, Salzman E W, De Sanctis R W, Coutts R D 1972 Prevention of venous thrombo-embolism following total hip replacement: warfarin vs dextran 40. Journal of American Medical Association 220: 1319–1322

Hellgren M. 1981 Thrombo-embolism and pregnancy. Studies on blood coagulation, fibrinolysis and treatment with heparin and antithrombin. M.D. thesis, Stockholm

Hellgren M, Blombäck M 1981 Blood coagulation and fibrinolysis in pregnancy, during delivery and in the puerperium. Gynecologic Obstetric Investigation 12: 141–154

Hellgren M, Hägnevik K, Blombäck M 1981 Heparin aerosol effects on blood coagulation and pulmonary function. Thrombosis Research 21: 493–502

Hellgren M, Nygards E B 1981 Blood coagulation and fibrinolysis in fertile women with previous thrombo-embolic complications and effects of venous occlusion. Thrombosis Research 24: 453–465

Hellgren M. Nygards E B 1982 Long-term therapy with subcutaneous heparin during pregnancy. Gynecologic Obstetric Investigation 13: 76–89

Hellgren M, Nygards H B, Robbe H 1982 Antithrombin III in late pregnancy. Acta obstetrica gynecologica scandinavica 61: 187–189

Hellgren M, Tenghorn L, Abildgaard U 1982 Pregnancy in women with congenital antithrombin III deficiency: experience of treatment with heparin and antithrombin. Gynecologic Obstetric Investigations 14: 127–141

Henderson S R, Lund C J, Creasman W Y 1972 Antepartum pulmonary embolism. American Journal of Obstetrics and Gynecology 112: 476–486

Hirsh J, Cade F J, O'Sullivan E F 1970 Clinical experience with anticoagulant therapy during pregnancy. British Medical Journal i: 270–273

Holzgreve W. Carey J C, Hall B D 1976 Warfarin-induced fetal abnormalities. Lancet ii: 914–915

Howell R, Fidler J, Letsky E, de Swiet M 1983 The risks of antenatal subcutaneous heparin prophylaxis: a controlled trial. British Journal of Obstetrics and Gynaecology 90: 1124–1128

Howie P W, Prentice C R M, Mallinson A C, Horne C H W, McNicol G P 1970 Effect of combined oestrogen-progestagen oral contraceptives, oestrogen and progestagen on antiplasmin and antithrombin activity. Lancet ii: 1329–1332

Hugo R, Von Hafter R, Hiller K F, Lochmuller H, Selbmann H K, Graeff H 1981 Prevention of deep-vein thrombosis in patients with gynaecological cancer undergoing radiotherapy. A comparison of calcium heparin and a semisynthetic analogue. Gebartsculfe und Frauenheilkunde 41: 179–183

Hull H, Hirsh J, Sackett D L, Powers P, Turpin A G G, Walker I 1977 Combined use of leg scanning and impedance plethysmography in suspected venous thrombosis. An alternative to venography. New England Journal of Medicine 296: 1495–1500

Ingram G I C, Brozovic M, Slater N G P 1982 Laboratory methods. In: Bleeding disorders — investigation and management, 2nd edn. Blackwell Scientific Publications, Oxford, ch 10 p 328

Jacques L B, Mahadoo J 1978 Pharmacodynamics and clinical effectiveness of heparin. Seminars in Thrombosis and Haemostasis 4: 298–325

Jacques L B, Mahadoo J, Kavanagh L W 1976 Intrapulmonary heparin. A new procedure for anticoagulant therapy. Lancet ii: 1157–1161

Johansson L, Hedner U, Nilsson I M 1978 Familial antithrombin III deficiency as pathogenesis of deep venous thrombosis. Acta medica scandinavica 201: 491–495

Kakkar V V, Lawrence D, Bentley P G, De Baas H A, Ward V P, Scully M F 1978 A comparative study of low doses of heparin and a heparin analogue in the prevention of postoperative deep vein thrombosis. Thrombosis Research 13: 111–122

Von Kaulla E, Von Kaulla K N 1970 Oral contraceptives and low antithrombin III activity. Lancet i: 36

Kerber I J, Warr O S II, Richardson R 1968 Pregnancy in a patient with a prosthetic mitral valve associated with a fetal anomoly attributed to warfarin sodium. Journal of the American Medical Association 203: 223–225

Kirklin J W 1981 The replacement of cardiac valves. New England Journal of Medicine 304: 291–292

Kline A, Hughes L E, Campbell H, Williams, A, Zlosnick J, Leach K G 1975 Dextran 70 in prophylaxis of thrombo-embolic disease after surgery — a clinically orientated randomised double blind trial. British Medical Journal ii: 109–112

Laerum F, Holm H A, Abildgaard U 1980 Anticoagulation and postphlebographic thrombosis. Lancet i: 1141–1142

Lane J L, Biggs R 1977 The natural inhibitors of coagulation: antithrombin III, heparin cofactor and antifactor Xa. In: Poller L (ed) Recent advances in blood coagulation. Churchill Livingstone, Edinburgh, p 123–139

Letsky E A, de Swiet M 1984 Thrombo-embolism in pregnancy and its management. British Journal of Haematology 57: No. 4

Limet R, Grondin C M 1977 Cardiac valve prostheses, anticoagulation and pregnancy. Annals of Thoracic Surgery 23: 337

Malcolm I D, Wigmore T A, Steinbrecher U P 1979 Heparin associated thrombocytopenia: low frequency in 104 patients treated with heparin of intestinal mucusal origin. Canadian Medical Association Journal 120: 1086–1088

Molino N. Belluardo C 1973 Considerazioni sull'uso dell' Esparina long-term nei cardiovasulopatici. Minerva cardiovasculogica 22: 553–557

Morris G K, Mitchell J R A 1978 Clinical management of venous thrombo-embolism. British Medical Bulletin 31: 169–175

Nagy H, Losonezy H, Szaksz I, Temesi C, Hegert K 1979 An analysis of clinical and laboratory data in patients with congenital antithrombin III (AtIII) deficiency. Acta medica academiae scientiarium hungaricae 36: 53–60

Negus D, Friedgood A, Derby S, Avery A, Wells B W 1980 Ultra-low-dose intravenous heparin in the prevention of postoperative deep vein thrombosis. Lancet i: 891–894

Oakley C M 1983 Pregnancy in patients with prosthetic heart valves. British Medical Journal 386: 1680–1682

Oakley C M, Doherty P 1976 Pregnancy in patients after valve replacement. British Heart Journal 38: 1140–1148

Orme M L'E et al 1977 May mothers given warfarin breast-feed their infants? British Medical Journal i: 1564–1565

Penn G B, Ross J W, Ashford A 1971 The effect of Arvin on pregnancy in the mouse and the rabbit. Toxicology and Applied Pharmacology 20: 460–473

Pettifor J M, Benson R 1875 Congenital malformations associated with the administration of oral anticoagulants during pregnancy. Journal of Pediatrics 86: 459–462

Poller L 1981 Oral anticoagulant therapy. In: Bloom A L, Thomas D P (eds) Haemostasis and thrombosis. Churchill Livingstone, Edinburgh, p 725–736

Poller L, Thomson J M 1964 Evidence for 'rebound' hypercoagulability after stopping anticoagulants. Lancet ii: 62–64

Pridmore B R, Murray K H, McAllen P M 1975 The management of anticoagulant therapy during and after pregnancy. British Journal of Obstetrics and Gynaecology 82: 740–744

Rhodes G R, Dixon R H, Silver D 1977 Heparin-induced thrombocytopenia: eight cases with thrombotic-haemorrhagic complications. Annals of Surgery 186: 752–758

Salzman E W, Rosenberg R D, Smith M H, Lindon J N, Favreau L 1980 Effect of heparin and heparin fractions on platelet aggregation. Journal of Clinical Investigation 65: 64–73

Shaul W L, Hall J G 1977 Multiple congenital anomalies associated with oral anticoagulants. American Journal of Obstetrics and Gynecology 127: 191–198

Sherman S, Hall B D 1972 Warfarin and fetal abnormality. Lancet i: 692

Simpson F G, Robinson P J, Bark M, Losowsky M S 1980 Prospective study of thrombo-phlebitis and 'pseudo thrombophlebitis'. Lancet i: 331–333

Spearing G, Frawer I, Turner G, Dixon G 1978 Long-term self-administered subcutaneous heparin in pregnancy. British Medical Journal ii: 1457–1458

de Swiet M, Bulpitt C.J, Lewis P J 1980 How obstetricians use anticoagulants in the prophylaxis of thrombo-embolism. Journal of Obstetrics and Gynaecology 1: 29–32

de Swiet M, Fidler J, Howell R, Letsky E A 1981 Thrombo-embolism in pregnancy. In: Jewell D P (ed) Advanced medicine 17: Pitman Medical, London, p 309–317

de Swiet M, et al 1983 Prolonged heparin therapy in pregnancy causes bone demineralisation (Heparin induced osteopenia) British Journal of Obstetrics and Gynaecology 90: 1129–1134

de Swiet M, Letsky E, Mellows H 1977 Drug treatment and prophylaxis of thrombo-embolism in pregnancy. In: Lewis P J (ed) Therapeutic problems in pregnancy. Medical and Technical Publishing Company Limited, Lancaster

Szekely P, Turner R, Snaith L 1973 Pregnancy and the changing pattern of rheumatic heart disease. British Heart Journal 35: 1293–1303

Taberner D A, Poller L, Burslem R W, Jones J B 1978 Oral anticoagulants controlled by the British comparative thromboplastin versus low-dose heparin in prophylaxis of deep vein thrombosis. British Medical Journal i: 272–274

Villasanta U 1965 Thrombo-embolic disease in pregnancy. American Journal of Obstetrics and Gynecology 93: 142–160

Whitfield L R, Lele A S, Levy G 1983 Effect of pregnancy on the relationship between concentration and anticoagulant action of heparin. Clinical Pharmacology and Therapeutics 34: 23–28

Wrigth C J. Jaques L B 1979 Heparin via the lung. Canadian Journal of Surgery 22: 317–319

3

Disseminated intravascular coagulation

The changes in the haemostatic system during pregnancy and the local activation of the clotting system during parturition carry a risk, not only of thrombo-embolism (see Ch. 2), but of disseminated intravascular coagulation (DIC). This results in consumption of clotting factors and platelets leading, in some cases, to severe uterine and sometimes generalised bleeding (Talbert & Blatt 1979).

The first problem with DIC is in its definition; it is never primary, but always secondary to some general stimulation of coagulation activity by release of procoagulant substances into the blood (Fig. 3.1). Hypothetical triggers of this process during pregnancy include the leaking into the maternal circulation of placental tissue fragments, amniotic fluid, incompatible red cells or bacterial products. There is a wide spectrum of manifestations (Table 3.1) ranging from a compensated state of no clinical manifestation but evidence of increased production and breakdown of coagulation factors, to the condition of massive uncontrollable haemorrhage with very low concentrations of plasma fibrinogen, pathological raised levels of fibrin degradation products (FDPs) and variable degrees of thrombocytopenia. Another confusing entity is what appears to be a transitory state of intravascular coagulation during normal labour, maximal at the time of birth (Gilabert et al 1978).

Fibrinolysis is stimulated by DIC and the FDPs resulting from the process interfere with the formation of firm fibrin clots, thus a vicious circle is established which results in further disastrous bleeding (Fig. 3.2).

Obstetric conditions classically associated with DIC include abruptio placentae, amniotic fluid embolism, septic abortion and intrauterine infection, retained dead fetus, hydatidiform mole,

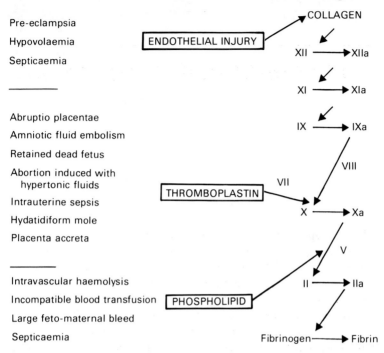

Fig. 3.1 Trigger mechanisms of DIC during pregnancy. Interactions of the trigger mechanisms occur in many of these obstetric complications.

placenta accreta, pre-eclampsia and eclampsia and prolonged shock from any cause (Fig. 3.1).

Despite the advances in obstetric care and highly developed blood transfusion services, haemorrhage still constitutes a major factor in maternal mortality and morbidity. While there have been many reports concerned with small series of patients or individual patients with coagulation failure during pregnancy, no significant controlled trials of the value of the many possible therapeutic measures have been undertaken. This is mainly because no one person or unit is likely to see sufficient cases to randomise them into groups in which the numbers would achieve statistical significance. Also the complex and variable nature of the conditions associated with DIC, which are often self-correcting and treated with a variety of measures, make it impossible to make an objective assessment of the published reports.

What follows is an outline of the strategy to deal with haemorrhage in the obstetric patient, arrived at by discussion of published reports

Table 3.1 Spectrum of severity of DIC relationship to specific complications in obstetrics

	Severity of DIC	In vitro findings	Obstetric condition commonly associated
Stage 1	Low grade compensated	FDPs ↑ Increased soluble fibrin complexes increased ratio $\dfrac{\text{factor VIII R: Ag}}{\text{factor VIIIC}}$	Pre-eclampsia Retained dead fetus
Stage 2	Uncompensated but no haemostatic failure	As above Plus fibrinogen ↓ platelets ↓ Factors V and VIII ↓	Small abruptio Severe pre-eclampsia
Stage 3	Rampant with haemostatic failure	Platelets ↓↓ Gross depletion of coagulation factors, particularly fibrinogen FDPs ↑	Abruptio placentae Amniotic fluid embolism Eclampsia

Rapid progression from stage 1 to stage 3 is possible unless appropriate measures are taken

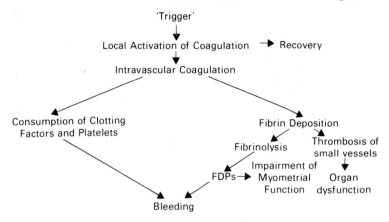

Fig. 3.2 Consequent effects following the stimulation of coagulation activity.

as well as the personal and collective experience of the staff at Queen Charlotte's Maternity Hospital.

Haematological management of the bleeding obstetric patient

The management of bleeding in an obstetric patient is an acute and frightening problem. There is no time to think and there should be a routine planned regimen of management in every maternity unit decided on by haematologist, physician, anaesthetist, obstetrician and nursing staff.

The management of haemorrhage is virtually the same, whether or not the bleeding is caused or augmented by coagulation failure. The clinical condition usually demands urgent treatment and there is no time to wait for results of coagulation factor assays or sophisticated tests of the fibrinolytic system activity for precise definition of the extent of haemostatic failure, although blood can be taken for this purpose and analysed at leisure once the emergency is over. Simple rapid tests recommended below will establish the competence or otherwise of the haemostatic system. In the vast majority of obstetric patients, coagulation failure results from a sudden transitory episode of DIC triggered by a variety of conditions (Fig. 3.1). Recovery will usually follow delivery of the patient provided that the blood volume is maintained and shock due to hypovolaemia is prevented. An efficiently acting myometrium postdelivery will stem haemorrhage from the placental site and measures taken to achieve a firm contracted uterus will obviously contribute one of the most important factors in preventing continuing massive blood loss.

As soon as there is any concern about a patient bleeding from any cause, approximately 15 ml of venous blood should be taken and delivered into a specific set of bottles kept in an emergency pack with a set of laboratory request forms previously made out which only require the patient's name and identification number added to them. This blood can be taken at the time of setting up an intravenous infusion if the patient does not already have one. It is essential that the blood should not be contaminated with even the smallest amount of heparin or the results obtained will be meaningless. If heparin has been used to set up an intravenous infusion then the blood *must* be taken from another site, however 'washed through' it is felt the line may be. The blood should be divided as follows:

1. **2.5 ml into EDTA for full blood count with emphasis on Hb, PCV and platelet count.**

2. **4.5 ml into citrate for coagulation screen.**

3. **2.0 ml into EACA for estimation of FDPs.**

4. **The rest, approximately 6.0 ml, into a plain tube for crossmatching.**

Useful rapid screening tests for haemostatic failure include the platelet count, partial thromboplastin time, or accelerated whole blood clotting time (which tests intrinsic coagulation), prothrombin time (which tests extrinsic coagulation), the thrombin time and estimation of fibrinogen (see Fig. 1.5, Ch. 1).

Elevation of FDPs is not specific to DIC and only confirms the diagnosis. The estimation is carried out on a clotted specimen delivered into EACA which prevents further fibrinolysis taking place in vitro. Of the tests of coagulation, probably the thrombin time, an estimation of the thrombin clottable fibrinogen in a citrated sample of plasma, is the most valuable overall rapid screen of haemostatic competence of coagulation factors. The normal thrombin time is around 10–15 seconds, and the fibrin clot formed is firm and stable. In the most severe forms of DIC there is no clottable fibrinogen in the sample, and no fibrin clot appears even after 2–3 minutes. Indication of severe DIC is obtained usually by a prolonged thrombin time with a friable clot which may dissolve on standing due to fibrinolytic substances present in the plasma (see Ch. 1, Tests of haemostatic function). A crude, but valuable rapid estimation of the fibrinogen level is obtained by a titre of the thrombin time test.

There is no point whatsoever in the obstetrician, anaesthetist or nursing staff wasting time trying to perform bedside whole blood clotting tests. Whole blood clotting normally takes up to 7 minutes and should be performed in clean tubes in a 37°C water bath with suitable controls and, at the end of the day, furnishes little information of practical value and only creates more panic. The valuable hands at the bedside are of more use doing the things they are trained to do in this emergency situation rather than wasting time performing a test which is time consuming, of little value or significance unless performed under strict control conditions, and will not contribute much, if anything, to management. The alerted laboratory worker will be able to provide significant results on which the obstetrician can act within half an hour at the most of receiving the specimen in the laboratory.

The tests referred to above are straightforward and should be available from any routine haematology laboratory; it is not necessary to have a high-powered coagulation laboratory to perform these simple screening tests.

Once the blood has been sent off to the laboratory for investigation, place two units of fresh, frozen plasma in a 37°C water bath to thaw. Fresh frozen plasma does not have to be crossmatched or given to patients of the same group from which it was taken, although it is preferable to use the same ABO and Rhesus group as the recipient if possible. While waiting for the plasma to thaw and for crossmatched blood, the circulation should be kept going with a plasma substitute. Treatment of severe haemorrhage must include prompt and adequate fluid replacement in order to avoid renal shutdown. If effective circulation is restored without too much delay FDPs will be cleared from the blood mainly by the liver, which will further aid restoration of normal haemostasis. *This is an aspect of management which is often not appropriately emphasised*

Use of plasma substitutes in the bleeding obstetric patient

There is much controversy around which plasma substitute to give to any bleeding patient. The remarks which follow are very much slanted towards the supportive laboratory management of *acute haemorrhage from the placental site* and should not be taken to apply to those situations in which hypovolaemia may be associated with severe hypoproteinaemia such as occurs in septic peritonitis, burns and bowel infarction. The choice lies between simple crystalloids, such as Hartmann's solution or Ringer lactate, and artificial colloids, such as dextrans, hydroxyethyl starch and gelatin solution or the very expensive preparations of human albumin (albuminoids). If crystalloids are used two to three times the volume of estimated blood loss should be administered because the crystalloid remains in the vascular compartment for a shorter time than colloids if renal function is maintained.

The infusion of plasma substitutes, i.e. plasma protein, dextran, gelatin and starch solutions may result in adverse reactions. Although the incidence of severe reactions is rare, they are diverse in nature, varying from allergic urticarial manifestation and mild fever to life-threatening anaphylactic reactions due to spasm of smooth muscle, with cardiac and respiratory arrest (Doenicke et al 1977).

Dextrans adversely affect platelet function, may cause pseudo-agglutination and interfere with interpretation of subsequent blood grouping and crossmatching tests. They are, therefore, contra-indicated in the woman who is bleeding due to a complication associated with pregnancy where there is a high chance of there being a serious haemostatic defect already. Dextrans are also associated with allergic anaphylactoid reactions. The anaphylactoid reactions accompanying infusion of dextrans are probably related to IgG and IgM antidextran antibodies which are found in high concentrations in all patients with severe reactions.

Albuminoids are thought to be associated less with anaphylactoid reactions but *they may be particularly harmful when transfused in the shocked patients by contributing to renal and pulmonary failure,* adversely affecting cardiac function and further impairing haemostasis (Cash 1981).

Many studies have suggested that the best way to deal with hypovolaemic shock initially is by transfusing simple balanced salt solutions (crystalloid) followed by red cells and fresh frozen plasma (Carey et al 1970, Moss 1972, Virgilio et al 1979). More recent work (Hauser et al 1980) has challenged this approach and suggests that albumin-containing solutions are superior to crystalloids for volume replacement in postoperative shocked patients with respiratory insufficiency. This aspect of the management of shocked patients with blood loss will remain controversial pending the results of further clinical trials. I advocate the use of a derivative of bovine gelatin — polygeline (Haemaccel) — as our first line fluid in resuscitation. It has a shelf-life of eight years and can be stored at room temperature. It is iso-oncotic and does not interfere with platelet function or subsequent blood grouping or crossmatching. Renal function is improved when it is administered in hypovolaemic shock. Haemaccel is generally considered to be nonimmunogenic and therefore does not trigger the production of antibodies in man, even on repeated challenge. The reactions which occur related to Haemaccel infusion are thought to be due to histamine release (Lorenz et al 1976), the incidence and severity of reactions being proportional to the extent of histamine release. There have been a few reports of severe reactions with bronchospasm and circulatory collapse, though rarely, and there has been one report of a fatality (Freeman 1979). Nevertheless, *whatever substitute is used it is only a stopgap until suitable blood component therapy can be administered.*

The use of whole blood and component therapy

Whole 'fresh' blood is not generally available in this country nowadays, because there is insufficient time to complete hepatitis surface antigen and blood grouping tests before it is released from the Transfusion Centre. To release it earlier than the usual 18–24 hours would increase the risk of transmitting viral B hepatitis and of serologically incompatible transfusions. Syphylis, cytomegalovirus (CMV) and Epstein Barr virus (EBV) are examples of other infections which may be transmitted in fresh blood but their viability diminishes rapidly on storage at 4°C. These infections, particularly in immunosuppressed or pregnant patients, can be particularly hazardous. Apart from the hazards of giving whole blood less than, say, 6–24 hours old, its use in this country today represents a serious waste of vitally needed components required for patients with specific isolated deficiencies. The use of fresh frozen plasma followed by bank red cells provides all the components, apart from platelets, present in whole fresh blood and allows the plasma from the freshly donated unit to be used to make the much needed blood components.

Plasma component therapy

Fresh frozen plasma (FFP): contains all the coagulation factors present in plasma obtained from whole blood within 6 hours of donation. Frozen rapidly and stored at −30°C, the factors are well preserved for at least 1 year but plasma stored at −20°C does degenerate and should be used within 6 months of preparation.

Freeze dried plasma: is prepared by pooling blood donations prior to dispensing and freezing and hence there is an increased risk of transmitting hepatitis. This product is also deficient in factors V and

VIII, but the advantage is that it can be stored in the dark below 25°C for up to 8 years. It can be of value in providing colloid in the management of surgical or traumatic haemorrhage.

Concentrated fibrinogen: should *not* be used in obstetric haemorrhage associated with DIC. The depletion of fibrinogen in these conditions is well known but undue importance is attributed to its lack which is part of a general consumptive coagulopathy. FFP provides abundant fibrinogen together with factors V, VIII which are also depleted and the coagulation inhibitor antithrombin III. Concentrated fibrinogen prepared from pooled donations carries a great risk of subsequent hepatitis and administration has been shown to result in a sharp fall in levels of antithrombin III, suggesting that the concentrates may aggravate intravascular coagulation (Bonnar 1981) by adding fuel to the fire. The concept of 'feeding the fire' by giving fresh frozen plasma to a patient who has DIC has not been proved. Although sometimes ineffective, such therapy has not been shown to do anything other than theoretical harm (Sharp 1977).

Platelets: an essential haemostatic component, are not present in FFP and their functional activity rapidly deteriorates in stored blood. The platelet count reflects both the degree of intravascular coagulation and the amount of bank blood transfused. A patient with persistent bleeding and very low platelet count (less than 20×10^9/l) may require concentrated platelets although in my limited experience I have never yet had to give them to achieve haemostasis. Indeed it has been suggested that platelet transfusions are more likely to do harm than good in this situation since most concentrates contain some damaged platelets which might in themselves provide a fresh trigger or mediator of DIC in the existing state (Sharp 1977). Platelet concentrates are specially prepared at the Transfusion Centre in packs using 3–5 donations of blood and have a shelf-life of only 72 hours.

Red cell transfusion

Crossmatched blood should be available within 40 minutes of the maternal specimen reaching the laboratory. If the woman has had all her antenatal care at the same hospital her blood group will be known and there is a good case for giving uncrossmatched blood of her same group should the situation warrant it, provided that blood has been properly processed at the Transfusion Centre. If the blood group is unknown uncrossmatched group O, Rhesus negative blood may be given if necessary. By this time laboratory screening tests of haemostatic function should be available. If these prove to be normal, but vaginal bleeding continues, the cause is nearly always trauma or bleeding from the placental site due to failure of the myometrium to contract. It is imperative that the source of bleeding, often an unsuspected uterine or genital laceration, be located and dealt with. Prolonged hypovolaemic shock or indeed shock from any cause, may also trigger off DIC and this may lead to haemostatic failure and further prolonged haemorrhage.

Stored whole blood, even under optimal conditions, undergoes certain deleterious changes. The oxygen affinity of red cells increases. Plasma ionic concentrations of potassium and hydrogen increase but these changes are not significant until after 4 days of shelf-life. Platelets deteriorate rapidly within the first 24 hours and after 72 hours they have lost all haemostatic function.

The activity of the labile coagulation factors V and particularly factor VIII decrease within the first 24 hours of donation. After 6 days storage microaggregates of platelets, white cells and fibrin form.

If the blood loss is replaced only by stored bank blood which is deficient in the labile clotting factors V and VIII and platelets then the circulation will rapidly become depleted in these essential components of haemostasis even if there is no DIC initially as the cause of haemorrhage. It is advisable to transfuse 1 unit of fresh frozen plasma for every 4–6 units of bank red cells administered.

It would seem sensible in any event, whatever the cause of bleeding, to change the initial plasma substitute and transfuse two units of fresh frozen plasma once it has thawed, while waiting for compatible blood to be available.

Finally, citrate used as an anticoagulant in transfused blood may complex calcium ions. Some centres recommend giving one ampoule (10 ml) of 10% calcium gluconate slowly over 10 minutes for every 6 units of blood infused. It would seem more sensible to check calcium levels routinely with the other electrolytes and treat only if indicated.

A spontaneous recovery from the coagulation defect is to be expected once the uterus is empty and well contracted, provided that blood volume is maintained by adequate replacement monitored by central venous pressure and urinary output.

Problems arise when bleeding is difficult to control and the woman has a low haemoglobin before blood loss, but this is unusual at term in a well-managed obstetric patient.

Clinicians may be helped in the decision of which replacement fluid to give in an obstetric emergency with the knowledge that very few bleeding patients die from lack of circulating red cells, the oxygen-carrying moiety of the blood. Death in the majority of cases results from poor tissue perfusion due to hypovolaemia. Every effort should be made to maintain a normal blood volume and restoration of red cell mass can be delayed until suitable compatibility tests have been performed and bleeding is at least partially controlled (Marshall & Bird 1983).

In normal circumstances the single most important component of haemostasis at delivery is contraction of the myometrium stemming the flow from the placental site. All the clotting factors and platelets in the world will not stop haemorrhage if the uterus remains flabby. Vaginal delivery will make a less severe demand on the haemostatic mechanism than delivery by caesarean section which requires the same haemostatic competence as any other major surgical procedure. Should DIC be established with the fetus in utero it is better to wait for spontaneous delivery, if possible, or stimulate vaginal delivery, avoiding episiotomy or other soft tissue damage, than to embark upon heroic surgical delivery.

Abruptio placentae

Premature separation of the placenta or abruptio placentae is the most frequent cause of coagulation failure in most patients. Many of the problems which confront the attendant in this situation are common to other conditions associated with DIC during pregnancy so that this will be used as the central focus to discuss some of the more controversial methods of management.

Abruptio placentae can occur without clinical warning in apparently healthy women as well as in those with established pre-eclampsia. It is possible that clinically silent placental infarcts may predispose to placental separation by causing low-grade abnormalities of the haemostatic system such as increased factor VIII consumption and raised FDPs (Redman 1979).

There is a wide spectrum in the severity of the haemostatic failure in this condition which appears to be related to the degree of placental separation. In some cases of a small abruptio, there is a minor degree of failure of the haemostatic processes and the fetus does not succumb (Table 3.1). When the uterus is tense and tender and no fetal heart can be heard, then separation and retroplacental bleeding are extensive. No guide to the severity of the haemorrhage or coagulation failure will be given by the amount of vaginal bleeding. Indeed, there may not be an external vaginal blood loss, even when the placenta is completely separated, the fetus dead, the circulating blood incoagulable and up to 5 litres of concealed blood loss. Haemostatic failure may be suspected if there is persistent oozing at the site of venipuncture or bleeding from the mucous membrane of mouth or nose. Simple rapid screening tests, as described in Chapter 1 and referred to below, will confirm the presence of DIC. There will be a low platelet count, greatly prolonged thrombin time, low fibrinogen, together with raised FDPs, due to secondary fibrinolysis stimulated by the intravascular deposition of fibrin (Estelles et al 1980). The mainstay of treatment is to maintain the circulating blood volume (see above). This not only prevents renal shutdown and further haemostatic failure caused by hypovolaemic shock, but helps clearance of FDPs which in themselves act as potent anticoagulants. It has also been suggested that FDPs inhibit myometrial activity and serious postpartum haemorrhage in women with abrupto placentae was found to be associated with high levels of FDP (Basu 1969, Sher 1977). There is some suggestion also that high levels of FDPs have a cardiotoxic effect. This important aspect of management of clearing products of coagulation from the circulation by maintaining the blood volume has not been appropriately emphasised (Pritchard 1973).

If the fetus is dead the aim should be prompt vaginal delivery avoiding soft tissue damage. Once correction of hypovolaemia is underway, measures to speed up delivery should be instituted. Amniotomy or, if this fails, prostaglandin or oxytocin stimulation can be used. There is no evidence that the use of oxytoxic agents aggravates thromboplastin release from the uterus (Bonnar 1978).

Following emptying of the uterus myometrial contraction will greatly reduce bleeding from the placental site and spontaneous correction of the haemostatic defect usually occurs shortly after delivery, if the measures recommended above have been taken. However postpartum haemorrhage is a not infrequent complication and is the commonest cause of death in abruptio placentae (DHSS 1982).

In cases where the abruptio is small and the fetus is still alive, prompt caesarean section may save the baby, if vaginal delivery is not imminent. Fresh frozen plasma, bank red cells and platelet concentrates should be available to correct the potentially severe coagulation defect in the maternal circulation (see above). In rare situations where vaginal delivery cannot be stimulated and haemorrhage continues, caesarean section may be indicated even in the presence of a dead fetus. In these circumstances normal haemostasis should be restored as far as possible by the administration of fresh frozen plasma and platelet concentrates, if necessary, as well as red cells before surgery is undertaken.

Despite extravasation of blood throughout the uterine muscle its function is not impaired and good contraction will follow the removal of fetus, placenta and retroplacental clot.

Hysterectomy should be avoided as delayed internal bleeding may occur. Regional anaesthesia or analgesia is of course contraindicated. Expansion of the lower limb vascular bed resulting from such regional blocking techniques can add to the problem of uncorrected hypovolaemia, and there is the additional hazard of bleeding into the epidural space (Bonnar 1981).

In recent years, heparin has been used to treat all kinds of disseminated intravascular coagulation, whatever their cause. There is, however, no objective evidence to demonstrate that its use in abruptio placentae decreases morbidity and mortality although anecdotal reports continue to suggest this (Thragarajah et al 1981). Very good results have been achieved without the use of heparin (Pritchard 1973). Its use, with an intact circulation, would be sensible and logical to break the vicious circle of DIC, but, in the presence of already defective haemostasis with a large bleeding placental site, it may prolong dangerous local and generalised haemorrhage (Feinstein 1982).

Treatment with antifibrinolytic agents such as EACA or Trasylol can result in blockage of small vessels of vital organs, such as the kidney or brain, with fibrin. They are therefore contraindicated, although Bonnar (1981) suggests that delayed severe and prolonged haemorrhage from the placental site several hours postdelivery may respond to their use if all other measures fail.

It has been suggested (Sher 1977) that Trasylol (aprotinin) may be helpful in the management of abruptio placentae, particularly in those cases with uterine inertia associated with high levels of FDPs. There is a high incidence (1.5%) of abruptio placentae in the obstetric admissions (18 000 per annum) at the Groote Scheur Obstetric Unit, Cape Town where the study was carried out.

Intravenous administration of Trasylol in 8 patients with abruptio placentae and uterine inertia, together with other prompt supportive measures, resulted in a rapid reco-ordination of uterine activity as well as a steady fall in serum FDP levels and a progressive rise in platelet count. The selection of the drug Trasylol as opposed to EACA depended on its alleged anticoagulant activity in addition to its well-known antifibrinolytic properties. An anticoagulant effect would make it a less hazardous agent in view of intravascular deposition of fibrin in vital organs and particularly useful in the management of haemorrhage due to DIC. However, in vitro studies indicate that very high concentrations are required to have any anticoagulant effect (Amris & Hilden 1968). Another study (Prentice et al 1970) showed high concentrations of Trasylol in vitro, appeared to inhibit the contact phase of coagulation only and the authors concluded that Trasylol would be a relatively weak anticoagulant in doses liable to be achieved in vivo. It would of course have no direct effect on the extrinsic coagulation pathway which is activated in the course of DIC due to abruptio placentae. However Nordstrom and colleagues (1968) showed that DIC in dogs, induced by injection of thromboplastin, was partially inhibited if they were treated prophylactically with Trasylol.

In recent years, the obstetric world as a whole appears unconvinced of the benefits of Trasylol in the treatment of DIC and abruptio placentae judging by many published reports.

Prompt supportive measures alone, maintaining central venous pressure and replacing blood loss together with essential coagulation factors, will of course result in reduction in FDPs. This will improve myometrial function and contribute to the return of healthy haemostasis.

One patient with recurrent abruptio placentae successfully treated with the fibrinolytic inhibitor tranexamic acid has been reported (Astedt & Nilsson 1978); the compound is related to epsilon amino caproic acid (EACA). Investigations on this woman suggested abnormally increased fibrinolytic activity in the 26th week of her third pregnancy. The previous two pregnancies had been complicated by abruptio placentae associated with a neonatal death and a stillbirth respectively. The intravenous administration of tranexamic acid following a small vaginal bleed resulted in restoration of normal coagulation status and the bleeding stopped; oral administration was continued. Another small bleed occurred at 33 weeks gestation, treated again with intravenous tranexamic acid. The eventual successful outcome of this pregnancy was attributed by the authors to the use of this agent, but there must have been many other variables involved.

Amniotic fluid embolism

Amniotic fluid embolism is very rare but is one of the most dangerous, if not the most dangerous, and untreatable conditions in obstetrics. The incidence has been estimated as between 1 in 8000 and 1 in 80 000 in various reports (see Morgan 1979) but the latter figure is probably nearer the true incidence. During the triennium 1976–78 in the British Isles 11 histologically confirmed and 8 suspected fatal cases occurred associated with 1 748 849 maternities. This gives an incidence of fatal amniotic fluid embolism of approximately 1 in 87 000 (DHSS 1982). The maternal mortality is very high: over 80% in most reports. An excellent recent review of 272 cases in the English literature reported that only 39 survived, giving a mortality rate of 86% (Morgan 1979).

Amniotic fluid embolism is said to occur most frequently in elderly multiparous patients with large babies at or near term following a short tumultuous labour associated with the use of uterine stimulants. However, the above review (Morgan 1979) did not substantiate this statement. The most recent Report of Confidential Enquiries into Maternal Deaths in England and Wales (DHSS 1982) confirmed that there were higher rates of mortality at older ages and higher parity but the relationship between violent contractions and rapid labour was less apparent.

There have been some reports of this complication of pregnancy occurring in different situations: in young primiparous women (see Morgan 1979) during the second trimester (Meier and Bowes 1983), in women undergoing legally induced terminations (Guidotti et al 1981), after evacuation of a missed abortion (Stromme & Fromke 1978) and even after deliberate termination of pregnancy (Cates et al 1981).

Amniotic fluid embolism is the most common cause of death in the immediate postpartum period (Herbert 1982).

The passage of amniotic fluid into the maternal circulation is thought to occur via the endocervical veins, the normal placental site, through uterine trauma at caesarean section or if the uterus ruptures. It is a prerequisite of amniotic fluid embolism that the fetal membranes be torn. Lethal amniotic fluid embolism is most commonly associated with small tears in the uterus, cervix or vagina which have not totally disrupted the wall (Rushton & Dawson 1982). This is not surprising since a complete tear would allow amniotic fluid to escape into the peritoneal cavity or to the vagina.

The clinical features associated with amniotic fluid embolism are respiratory distress, cyanosis, cardiovascular collapse, haemorrhage and coma. Although coagulation failure occurs rapidly the presenting clinical feature is sudden extreme shock with cyanosis due to an almost complete shutdown of the pulmonary circulation

76

followed by the onset of intractable uterine bleeding. The coagulation abnormalities are ascribed to the thromboplastic activity of amniotic fluid (Courtney & Allington 1972, Yaffe et al 1977). Massive intravascular coagulation occurs and consumption of the clotting factors can be almost total (Bonnar 1981). Platelet fibrin thrombi are formed and are trapped within the pulmonary blood vessels and profound shock follows accompanied by respiratory distress and cyanosis. There is a high mortality at this stage from a combination of respiratory and cardiac failure; if the mother survives long enough the effect of massive intravascular coagulation will invariably follow with bleeding from venipuncture sites and severe haemorrhage from the placental site after delivery (Gregory & Clayton 1973).

Until recently confirmation of diagnosis could only be made at autopsy by finding histological evidence of amniotic fluid and fetal tissue within the substance of the maternal lungs, with or without identification of the portal of entry in the placenta or uterine wall (Rushton & Dawson 1982). It is therefore difficult to assess the value of therapeutic measures suggested in the few reports which have appeared of successful management of a clinical syndrome diagnosed clinically as amniotic fluid embolism (Bonnar 1973, Skjodt 1965, Chung & Merkatz 1973, Resnik et al 1976). More recent techniques of diagnosis include detection of squamous cells and lanugo hair on cytological examination of blood aspirated through a Swan-Ganz catheter and detection of squamous cells in maternal sputum (Herbert 1982). A recent report (Dolynuick et al 1983) describes a case in which the diagnosis of amniotic fluid embolism was made using these techniques and the patient survived. In a 19-year-old primigravida acute respiratory failure developed following caesarean section; fragments of vernix caseosa were identified in a pulmonary artery blood sample obtained through a Swan-Ganz catheter. The patient received intensive supportive care and recovered completely. A word of warning concerning the management of cardiorespiratory failure associated with amniotic fluid embolism is necessary here. This condition is similar to pulmonary embolism but there is also profound haemorrhage and too rigorous attempts at maintenance of the circulation, as recommended above for other conditions associated with DIC, may result in cardiac failure. There should be careful monitoring of the central venous pressure to avoid cardiac overload; the object is to sustain the circulation while the intravascular thrombin in the lungs is cleared by the naturally stimulated intense fibrinolytic response of the endothelium of the pulmonary vessels.

Measures to stimulate uterine contraction to reduce blood loss from the placental site are important in maintaining the blood volume. If bleeding from the placental site can be controlled by stimulation of uterine contraction then the logical treatment is carefully monitored transfusion of fresh frozen plasma and packed red cells with heparin administration and if indicated positive pressure ventilation (Bonnar 1981). It is obviously essential that a competent intensive care unit is immediately available to any obstetric service to deal promptly with this rare but often lethal complication of pregnancy.

Retention of a dead fetus

There is a gradual depletion of maternal coagulation factors following intrauterine death (IUD) but the changes are not usually detectable until after 3–4 weeks (Hodgkinson et al 1964). Thromboplastic substances released from the dead fetal tissues into the maternal circulation are thought to be the trigger for DIC, which occurs in about one-third of patients who retain the dead fetus for such an interval (Pritchard 1959). There is depletion of fibrinogen, factor VIII and platelets, together with elevation of FDPs. Gross increase of soluble fibrin/fibrinogen complexes amounting to 25% of the total fibrinogen in association with a dead fetus has been described (Hafter & Graeff 1975). Happily, around 80% of pregnant women will go into spontaneous labour within three weeks of intrauterine fetal death and in modern obstetric practice, labour is usually induced within 3–4 weeks in those who do not.

Rupture of the membranes is recommended once labour is established in patients with an IUD as amniotic fluid embolism has been known to occur (Bonnar 1978).

If the screening tests previously described indicate that there is defective haemostasis the coagulation factors should be restored to normal before delivery is attempted. Where the circulation is intact heparin is the logical treatment to check the activation of the coagulation systems. Intravenous infusion of 1000 i.u. heparin hourly for up to 48 hours is usually sufficient to restore the number of platelets, and the level of fibrinogen and factors V and VIII to normal (Bonnar 1978). The heparin should then be discontinued and onset of labour stimulated. There should be a plentiful supply of compatible red cells and fresh frozen plasma standing by to treat any haemorrhage at placental separation promptly. Should the patient go into spontaneous labour while heparin is being administered, the infusion should be stopped. It is not necessary to neutralise the heparin with protamine sulphate unless the patient is bleeding. *There is no rational basis for the use of fibrinolytic inhibitors in the management of the patient with coagulation failure associated with a retained dead fetus.* The increased fibrinolytic activity is secondary to DIC and the defective haemostasis will be corrected by the powerful anticoagulant effect of heparin in the presence of an intact circulation before the onset of labour.

Abortion and DIC

Changes in haemostatic components consistent with DIC have been demonstrated in patients undergoing abortion induced with hypertonic solutions of saline and urea (Spivak et al 1972, Van Royen 1974, MacKenzie et al 1975, Grundy & Craven 1976). The stimulus appears to be the release of tissue factor into the maternal circulation from the placenta, which is damaged by the hypertonic solutions. DIC in association with late cervical dilatation and evacuation procedures has also been described (Davis 1972) as well as in association with prostaglandin and oxytocin methods (Savage 1982). The risk of DIC was increased five times in women receiving oxytocin while undergoing induced saline abortions (Cohen & Ballard 1974), but in another study the risk of DIC in women given urea plus prostaglandin or oxytocin was only one-quarter of that for women receiving saline alone (Burkman et al 1977). Haemorrhage may be massive and has resulted in maternal deaths. Prompt restoration of the blood volume and transfusions with red cells and fresh frozen plasma as described above should resolve the situation which, once the uterus is empty, is self-limiting.

Intrauterine infection

Endotoxic shock associated with septic abortion or intrauterine infection pre- or post delivery can trigger DIC (Graeff et al 1976, Steichele & Herschlein 1968); infection with Gram negative micro-organisms is the usual finding. Fibrin is deposited in the microvasculature due to endothelial damage by the endotoxin and secondary red cell intravascular haemolysis with characteristic fragmentation, so-called microangiopathic haemolysis is characteristic of the condition.

The patient is unusually alert, flushed, has a rapid pulse and low blood pressure. Transfusion, unlike other obstetric emergencies complicated by DIC, has little or no effect on the hypotension. Some few centres in Europe have used heparinisation in the management of septic abortion and have claimed a decrease in mortality (Bonnar 1978). In the situation where the uterus is empty and contracted, hence no undue risk of severe bleeding from the placental site, and laboratory evidence indicates a consumptive coagulopathy, heparin may be useful as part of the management (Clarkson et al 1969).

As stated previously DIC is always a secondary phenomenon and the mainstay of management is to remove the initiating stimulus if possible; in the above situation elimination of the uterine infection remains the most important aspect of management. Claims that therapy with heparin has decreased maternal mortality in septic abortion are open to doubt and the use of heparin remains controversial (Beller & Uszynski 1974).

It is of interest that the mortality of DIC associated with placental abruption is less than 1% (Pritchard & Brekken 1967), whereas that associated with infection and shock is 50–80% (Mant & King 1979). The mortality rate reported in series of patients with DIC due to various aetiologies is 50–85% and the wide variation probably reflects the mortality rate of the underlying disorder, not of DIC per se (Feinstein 1982). Indeed, DIC itself probably contributes little to overall mortality, relative to the underlying and provoking cause.

Purpura fulminans

This rare complication sometimes occurs during the puerperium, precipitated by Gram negative septicaemia. Extensive haemorrhage occurs into the skin in association with DIC. The underlying mechanism is unknown but there appears to be an acute activation of the clotting system resulting in the deposition of fibrin thrombi within blood vessels of the skin and other organs (McGibbon 1982). The extremities and face are usually involved first, the purpuric patches having a jagged and erythematous border, which can be shown histologically to be the site of a leucocytoclastic vasculitis. Rapid enlargement of the lesions, which become necrotic and gangrenous, is associated with shock tachycardia and fever. Without treatment the mortality rate is high and in those who survive major amputation may be necessary. The laboratory findings are those of DIC with a leucocytosis. In this situation, treatment with heparin should be started as soon as the diagnosis is apparent. It will prevent further consumption of platelets and coagulation factors. It should always be remembered however that bleeding from any site in the presence of defective coagulation factors will be aggravated by the use of heparin.

Survival in purpura fulminans is currently much improved because of better supportive treatment for the shocked patient, effective control of the triggering infection, together with heparin therapy.

Acute fatty liver of pregnancy (AFLP)

This is a rare complication of pregnancy and included in this section because it is often, if not always, associated with variable degrees of DIC which contributes significantly to its morbidity and mortality (Feinstein 1982). First identified by Sheehan (1940) as a separate entity, there have now been about 90 patients documented in the English literature (Burroughs et al 1982) and probably less than 150 cases in the world literature (Hague et al 1983). The salient histological factors on which the diagnosis is ultimately based are the presence of fat in small vacuoles in centrilobular hepatocytes while a ring of normal hepatocytes remains around the portal systems without any evidence of cellular necrosis (Davies et al 1980). Renal failure with tubular necrosis is a common association (Rushton & Dawson 1982). The aetiology of this rare condition remains unknown.

A similar picture outside pregnancy can be produced by prolonged administration of tetracyclines and has been reported following intravenous administration of high doses of this drug during pregnancy (Schultz et al 1963). A similar condition occurs in ewes during the latter two-fifths of pregnancy, associated with multiple pregnancy or occasionally one large single lamb. It is known as pregnancy toxaemia of sheep or twin lamb disease (Ferris et al 1969)

Clinical presentation is typically during the last trimester with sudden onset of malaise, nausea, repeated vomiting and abdominal pain followed by jaundice. Haematemesis often occurs (Burroughs et al 1982) and is part of a bleeding diathesis due to thrombocytopenia, consumption coagulopathy and defects of coagulation factor synthesis (Anon 1983).

The fetus is usually stillborn and following delivery, the mother lapses into deeper coma associated with progressive hepatic and renal failure. The maternal mortality is between 75 and 85% and the fetal mortality is around 85% (Burroughs et al 1983). There are some few reports of this condition presenting in the puerperium (Anon 1983).

Diagnosis during life has usually been made on clinical grounds alone in the past because the severe coagulation defect precludes liver biopsy. Even at postmortem the acute fatty liver may well go undiagnosed unless the liver is carefully examined histologically ·using specific stains. An apparently normal liver to naked eye inspection may show severe fatty infiltration on microscopic examination (Anon 1983).

Proteinuria, hypertension and oedema are frequent accompanying features (Burroughs et al 1982) but pre-eclampsia is a much more common complication of pregnancy than AFLP. Thus, with the possibility of the missed histological diagnosis, the validity of statistics concerning the incidence of AFLP must be questioned. The most recent Confidential Enquiries into Maternal Deaths in England and Wales (DHSS 1982) attributed 29 deaths to hypertensive diseases of pregnancy of which 21 were associated with cerebral haemorrhage, cerebral oedema, DIC and hepato-renal failure, all of which are well recognised features of AFLP. In the same period only 7 deaths were attributed to liver disorders. The distinction between eclampsia and AFLP may not be as clear as has been previously assumed: they may represent different clinical exoressions of the same underlying disorder, and deaths due to AFLP may have been underestimated. Transient deficiencies of the urea cycle enzymes have been described in AFLP and many such cases follow an acute infective illness. In these two respects the condition resembles Reyes syndrome (Weber et al 1979).

It has been suggested that metabolic failure is precipitated by acute stress acting on a susceptible liver which is already dealing with the demands of the third trimester (Hague et al 1983). Analysis of total reports in the literature and individual series, show a high incidence of male fetuses and of twins associated with AFLP (Burroughs et al 1982, Hague et al 1983, Anon 1983).

Most observers agree that prompt delivery of the fetus offers the best chance of survival of both mother and child. Both caesarean section and induction of labour led to a lower than expected maternal and fetal mortality in a series of 12 patients reported from the Royal Free Hospital (Burroughs et al 1982). This being so, early accurate diagnosis would seem to be a prerequisite for improving survival of both mother and child.

Most patients have prodromal symptoms for at least one week before jaundice develops. The Royal Free series drew attention to a characteristic blood picture of neutrophilia, thrombocytopenia and normoblasts. Some of the blood films available for review showed basophilic stippling and giant platelets and the authors suggest that these appearances might help towards an early diagnosis of AFLP (Burroughs et al 1982). However, these features are not specific to AFLP and may be seen in any condition of additional stress on a bone marrow already working to capacity in the last trimester of pregnancy.

There should be a high order of suspicion when nausea and vomiting occur late in pregnancy, particularly if accompanied by abdominal pain and heartburn and associated with twins. This combination warrants immediate admission to hospital for investigation and observation. Further studies are required to establish the value of liver function tests, uric acid levels, amino acid profiles and examination of the blood film to achieve an early diagnosis of AFLP. Biospy of the liver obtained before delivery would be valuable in establishing the diagnosis but is often precluded because of the severe haemostatic defect. It has not been established yet whether using computerised axial tomography would aid diagnosis, as has been suggested in other conditions with fatty liver (Bydder et al 1980).

In AFLP the haemostatic defect is frequently extended, probably due to prolonged activation of coagulation combined with very low or even undetectable antithrombin III levels (Feinstein 1982): antithrombin III concentrate has been used in the successful management of such a patient (Laursen et al 1981) and the replacement of antithrombin III with plasma or concentrate to shorten the period of DIC and thereby decrease morbidity and mortality has been suggested (Feinstein 1982).

At the present time the clinical problem of AFLP remains that of early diagnosis since prompt delivery seems to be the specific management which limits progression of the disease and decreases both maternal and fetal mortality.

REFERENCES

Amris C J, Hilden M 1968 Anticoagulant effects of Trasylol: in vitro and in vivo studies. Annals of the New York Academy of Sciences 146: 612–624

Anon 1983 Acute fatty liver of pregnancy: Lancet i; 339

Astedt B, Nilsson I M 1976 Recurrent abruptio placentae treated with the fibrinolytic inhibitor tranexamic acid. British Medical Journal i: 756–757

Basu H K 1969 Fibrinolysis and abruptio placentae. Journal of Obstetrics and
Gynaecology of the British Commonwealth 76: 481–496
Beller F K, Uszynski M 1974 Disseminated intravascular coagulation in
pregnancy. Clinics in Obstetrics and Gynecology 17: 264–278
Bonnar J 1973 Blood coagulation and fibrinolysis in obstetrics. Clinics in
Haematology 2: 213–233
Bonnar J 1978 Haemorrhagic disorders during pregnancy in perinatal coagulation.
In: Hathaway W E, Bonnar J (eds) Monographs in neonataology, Grune &
Stratton Inc, New York
Bonnar J 1981 Haemostasis and coagulation disorders in pregnancy. In: Bloom A
L, Thomas D P (eds) Haemostasis and thrombosis, Churchill Livingstone,
Edinburgh p 454–471
Burkman R T, Bell W R, Atienza M F, King T M 1977 Coagulopathy with
midtrimester induced abortion. Association with hyperosmolar urea
administration. American Journal of Obstetrics and Gynecology 127: 533–536
Burroughs A K, Seong N G, Dojcinoov D M, Scheuer P J, Sherlock S V P 1982
Idiopathic acute fatty liver of pregnancy in 12 patients. Quarterly Journal of
Medicine 51: 481–497
Bydder G M, Kreel L, Chapman R W G, Harry D, Sherlock S 1980 Accuracy of
computerised tomography in diagnosis of fatty liver. British Medical Journal 281:
1042–1044
Carey L C, Cloumer C T, Lowery B D 1970 The use of balanced electrolyte
solution for resuscitation. In: Fox Nahas (ed) Body fluid replacement in the
surgical patient, Grune & Stratton, New York
Cash J 1981 Blood replacement therapy. In: Bloom A L, Thomas D P (eds)
Haemostasis and thrombosis, Churchill Livingstone, Edinburgh
Cates W Jr, Boyd C, Halvorson-Boyd G, Holck S, Gilchrist T F 1981 Death from
amniotic fluid embolism and disseminated intravascular coagulation after a
curettage abortion. American Journal of Obstetrics and Gynecology 141:
346–348
Chung A F, Merkatz I R 1973 Survival following amniotic fluid embolism with
early heparinisation. Obstetrics and Gynecology 42: 809–814
Clarkson A R, Sage R E, Lawrence J R 1969 Consumption coagulopathy and
acute renal failure due to Gram negative septicaemia after abortion. Complete
recovery with heparin therapy. Annals of Internal Medicine 70: 1191–1199
Cohen E, Ballard G A 1974 Consumptive coagulopathy associated with
intraamniotic saline instillation and the effect of intravenous oxytocin.
Obstetrics and Gynaecology 43: 300–303
Courtney L D, Allington M 1972 Effect of amniotic fluid on blood coagulation.
British Journal of Haematology 29: 353–356
Davies M H et al 1980 Acute liver disease with encephalopathy and renal failure
in late pregnancy and the early puerperium. A study of fourteen patients.
British Journal of Obstetrics and Gynaecology 87: 1003–1014
Davis G 1972 Midtrimester abortion. Late dilation and evacuation and DIC.
Lancet ii: 1026
Department of Health and Social Security 1982 Report on Health and Social
Subjects 26. Report on Confidential Enquiries into Maternal Deaths in England
and Wales 1976–78. Her Majesty's Stationery Office, London
Doenicke A, Grote B, Lorenz W 1977 Blood and blood substitutes. British
Journal of Anaesthesia 49: 681–688
Dolyniuk M, Orfei E, Vania H, Karlman R, Tomich P 1983 Rapid diagnosis of
amniotic fluid embolism. Obstetrics and Gynecology 61: supplement No. 3
28S–30S
Estelles A, Aznar J, Gilabert J 1980 A quantitative study of soluble fibrin
monomer complexes in normal labour and abruptio placentae. Thrombosis
Research 18: 513–519

Feinstein D I 1982 Diagnosis and management of disseminated intravascular coagulation: the role of heparin therapy. Blood 60: 284–287

Ferris T F, Herdson P B, Dunhill M S, Lee M R 1969 Toxaemia of pregnancy in sheep: a clinical physiological and pathological study. Journal of Clinical Investigation 48: 1643–1655

Freeman M 1979 Fatal reaction to Haemaccel. Anaesthesia 34: 341–343

Gilabert J, Aznar J, Parrilla J, Reganon E, Vila V, Estelles A 1978 Alteration in the coagulation and fibrinolysis system in pregnancy, labour and puerperium, with special reference to a possible transitory state of intravascular coagulation during labour. Thrombosis and Haemostasis 40: 387–396

Graeff H, Ernst E, Bocaz J A 1978 Evaluation of hypercoagulability in septic abortion. Haemostasis 5: 285–294

Gregory M G, Clayton E M J 1973 Amniotic fluid embolism. Obstetrics and Gynecology 42: 236–244

Grundy M F B, Craven E R 1976 Consumption coagulopathy after intra-amniotic urea. British Medical Journal ii: 677–678

Guidotti R J, Grimes D A, Cates W Jr. 1981 Fatal ambiotic fluid embolism during legally induced abortion. United States, 1972 to 1978. American Journal of Obstetrics and Gynecology 141: 257–261

Hafter R, Graeff H 1975 Molecular aspects of defibrination in a reptilase treated case of 'dead fetus syndrome'. Thrombosis Research 7: 391–399

Hague W M, Fenton D W, Duncan S L B, Slater D N 1983 Acute fatty liver of pregnancy. Journal of the Royal Society of Medicine 76: 652–661

Hauser C J, Shoemaker W C, Turpin I, Goldberg S J 1980 Oxygen transport responses to colloids and crystalloids in critically ill surgical patients. Surgica gynecologica obstetrica 159: 181–186

Herbert W N P 1982 Complications of the immediate puerperium. Clinical Obstetrics and Gynecology 25: 219–232

Hodgkinson C R, Thompson R J, Hodari A A 1964 Dead fetus syndrome. Clinical Obstetrics and Gynecology 7: 349–358

Laursen B, Mortensen J Z, Frost L, Hansen K B 1981 Disseminated intravascular coagulation in hepatic failure treated with antithrombin III. Thrombosis Research 22: 701–704

Lorenz W et al 1976 Histamine release in human subjects by modified gelatin (Haemaccel) and dextran: an explanation for anaphylactoid reactions observed under clinical conditions. British Journal of Anaesthesai 48: 151–165

McGibbon D H 1982 Dermatological purpura. In: Ingram G I C, Brozovic M, Slater N G P (eds) Bleeding disorders — investigation and management, Blackwell Scientific Publications, Oxford

MacKenzie I Z et al 1975 Coagulation changes during second trimester abortion induced by intra-amniotic prostaglandin E_2 and hypertonic solutions. Lancet ii: 1066–1069

Mant M J, King E G 1979 Severe acute disseminated intravascular coagulation. A reappraisal of its pathophysiology, clinical significance and therapy based on 47 patients. American Journal of Medicine 67: 557–563

Marshall M, Bird T 1983 Blood loss and replacement. Edward Arnold (pubs) Ltd, London

Meier P R, Bowes W A 1983 Amniotic fluid embolus-like syndrome presenting in the second trimester of pregnancy. Obstetrics and Gynecology 61: Supplement No.3, 31S–34S

Morgan M 1979 Amniotic Fluid Embolism. Anaesthesia 34: 20–32

Moss G 1972 An argument in favour of electrolyte solutions for early resuscitation. Surgical clinics in North America 52: 3–17

Nordström S, Blömback B, Blömback M, Olsson P, Zettequist E 1968 Experimental investigations on the antithromboplastic and antifibrinolytic activity of Trasylol. Annals of the New York Academy of Sciences 146: 701–714

Coagulation Problems During Pregnancy

Prentice C R M, McNicol G P, Douglas A 1970 Studies on the anticoagulant action of aprotinin ('Trasylol'). Thrombosis et Diathesis Haemorrhagica 24: 265–272

Pritchard J A 1959 Fetal death in utero. Obstetrics and Gynecology 14: 573–580

Pritchard J A 1973 Haematological problems associated with delivery, placental abruption, retained dead fetus and amniotic fluid embolism. Clinics in Haematology 2: 563–586

Pritchard J A, Brekken A L 1967 Clinical and laboratory studies on severe abruptio placentae. American Journal of Obstetrics and Gynecology 97: 681–695

Redman C W G 1979 Coagulation problems in human pregnancy. Postgraduate Medical Journal 55: 367–371

Resnik R, Swartz W H, Plumer M H, Bernirske K, Stratthaus M E 1976 Amniotic fluid embolism with survival. Obstetrics and Gynecology 47: 395–298

Van Royen E A 1974 Haemostasis in human pregnancy and delivery. M.D. thesis. University of Amsterdam

Rushton D I, Dawson I M P 1982 The maternal autopsy. Journal of Clinical Pathology 35: 909–921

Savage W 1982 Abortion: Methods and sequelae. British Journal of Hospital Medicine 27: 364–384

Schultz J, Adamson J, Workman W, Norman T 1963 Fatal liver disease after intravenous administration of tetracycline in high dose. New England Journal of Medicine 269: 999–1004

Sharp A A 1977 Diagnosis and management of disseminated intravascular coagulation. British Medical Bulletin 33: 265–272

Sheehan H 1940 The pathology of acute yellow atrophy and delayed chloroform poisoning. Journal of Obstetrics and Gynaecology of the British Empire 47: 49–62

Sher G 1977 Pathogenesis and management of uterine inertia complicating abruptio placentae with consumption coagulopathy. American Journal of Obstetrics and Gynecology 129: 164–170

Skjodt P 1965 Amniotic fluid embolism — a case investigated by coagulation and fibrinolysis studies. Acta obstetrica gynecologica scandinavica 44: 437–457

Spivak J L, Sprangler D B, Bell W R 1972 Defibrination after intra-amniotic injection of hypertonic saline. New England Journal of Medicine 287: 321–323

Steichele D F, Herschlein H J 1968 Intravascular coagulation in bacterial shock. Consumption coagulopathy and fibrinolysis after febrile abortion. Med Welt 1: 24–30

Stromme W B, Fromke V L 1979 Amniotic fluid embolism and disseminated intravascular coagulation after evacuation of missed abortion. Obstetrics and Gynecology 52: 76S–80S

Talbert I M, Blatt P M 1979 Disseminated intravascular coagulation in obstetrics. Clinics in Obstetrics and Gynecology 22: 889–900

Thragarajah S, Wheby M S, Jarn R, May H V, Bourgeois J, Kitchin J D 1981 Disseminated intravascular coagulation in pregnancy. The role of heparin therapy. Journal of Reproductive Medicine 26: 17–24

Tuck C S 1972 Amniotic fluid embolus. Proceedings of the Royal Society of Medicine 65: 94–95

Virgilio R J, et al 1979 Crystalloid versus colloid resuscitation: is one better? Surgery 85: 129–139

Weber F L, Snodgrass P J, Powell D E, Rao P, Huffman S L, Brady P G 1979 Abnormalities of hepatic mitochondrial urea-cycle, enzyme activities and hepatic ultrastructure in acute fatty liver of pregnancy. Journal of Laboratory and Clinical Medicine 94: 27–41

Webster J, Rees A J, Lewis P J, Hensby C N 1980 Prostacyclin deficiency in haemolytic uraemic syndrome. British Medical Journal 281: 271

Yaffe H, Eldor A, Hornshtein E, Sadovsky E 1977 Thromboplastin activity in amniotic fluid during pregnancy. Obstetrics and Gynecology 50: 454–456

4

Obstetric conditions commonly associated with abnormal changes in the haemostatic response to pregnancy

Pregnancy hyptertension and impaired fetal growth

Both of these conditions may be associated with quite marked changes in the normal physiological response of the haemostatic mechanisms during pregnancy. Whether these changes are primary or secondary to a basic trigger mechanism or mechanisms is a matter for debate. What follows is an account of the changes in vascular response, coagulation and fibrinolysis known to occur, speculation as to what may be their cause and an account of some of the attempts to alter the course of these conditions by correcting the haemostatic defects. In no way is this section intended to be a comprehensive review of these very complicated and unresolved areas of obstetrics care but rather to highlight the role of haemostatic factors in the pathogenesis of pregnancy hypertension and intrauterine fetal growth retardation: (IUGR).

I believe that both pre-eclampsia and late fetal growth retardation are an expression of intravascular coagulation which, in turn, is always a secondary phenomenon. Thus attempts to lower blood pressure or improve fetal growth by treating the haemostatic defect without removing the underlying cause (presently unknown in both cases) largely are bound to end in failure. However no account of pathological haemostasis during pregnancy would be complete without at least some discussion of these very speculative areas of pregnancy hypertension and impaired fetal growth.

Haemostasis and pre-eclampsia

The aetiology of pre-eclampsia is unknown; indeed so many hypotheses have been produced as possible basic trigger mechanisms that it has been labelled 'the disease of theories' for more than 50 years (McGillivray 1981). However, considerable evidence has accumulated over the past decade that DIC regularly plays a part in at least the pathogenesis of the condition (Howie 1977, Bonnar & Sheppard 1981, McKay 1981). Immune mechanisms have also been shown to play a part and are seemingly of relevance in respect to the incidence in primigravidae.

The immunological and haemostatic systems normally interact at many levels, being in dynamic equilibrium with each other with respect to platelet function, fibrin degradation and fibrinolysis thus maintaining a satisfactory blood supply to vital organs.

A concept of abnormal platelet and coagulation activity, perhaps triggered by immune mechanisms, could explain many of the features of pre-eclampsia and eclampsia by leading to obstruction of blood supply to the placenta, kidney, liver and brain.

Whatever the trigger there are certain changes in the haemostatic mechanisms which occur regularly in pre-eclampsia (see Table 4.1).

Table 4.1 Haemostatic changes observed in pre-eclampsia and intrauterine growth retardation

Prostacyclin	Decreased	
Platelets	Increased consumption	
	Decreased lifespan	
	Decreased 5HT	
Factor VIII	Increased consumption	
		Factor VIII R.Ag
	Increased ratio	——————————
		Factor VIII C
Soluble fibrin complexes	Increased	
Fibrin degradation products	Increased in serum and urine	
Plasminogen activator	Decreased	

Prostacyclin in pre-eclampsia

Prostacyclin (PGI_2) is the principal prostanoid synthesised by blood vessels. It is a powerful inhibitor of platelet aggregation and a vasodilator which is particularly active on the venous side of the circulation. It has been suggested that there is a balance between the production of thromboxane by the platelet and the production of prostacyclin by the vessel wall that that this dynamic equilibrium helps to control the tendency of platelets to aggregate (Moncada & Vane 1979) and that prostacyclin is the potent local substance produced continuously by healthy vascular tissue protecting the endothelial cells against platelet deposition (Moncada & Vane 1981) (see Ch. 1). A deficiency of prostacyclin production has been proposed in conditions associated with intravascular platelet consumption such as haemolytic uraemic syndrome and thrombotic thrombocytopenia purpura (Remuzzi et al 1978, Remuzzi et al 1980b). It has also been suggested that a relative deficiency of prostacyclin might be a central defect in pre-eclampsia (Lewis 1982).

The first identification of prostacyclin in human placenta was made by Myatt & Elder (1977) and its stable metabolite 6-OXO $PGF_{1\alpha}$ can be detected and measured in amniotic fluid during late pregnancy (Mitchell et al 1979). Myometrium synthesises prostacyclin and its capacity to do so increases with advancing gestation (Bamford et al 1980).

Fetal blood vessels produce prostacyclin in the same way as adult blood vessels (Downing et al 1982) while umbilical cord arteries synthesise more prostacyclin than blood vessels from normal adults. It is the high capacity of fetal and placental blood vessels to produce prostacyclin and therefore dilate which has been suggested as the mechanism whereby the fetal circulation is able to maintain a low arterial pressure and facilitate blood flow in the face of a high cardiac output (Remuzzi et al 1979). Indeed a direct relation was shown between blood flow in the fetus and umbilical prostacyclin production by Mäkilä et al (1983). The capacity of the components of the uteroplacental unit to produce prostacyclin must contribute prostacyclin to the maternal circulation and high levels of 6-OXO-$PGF_{1\alpha}$ have been found there in normal women during late pregnancy (Lewis et al 1980).

In pre-eclampsia there is generalised vasoconstriction and a relative decrease in the maternal intravascular volume; increased platelet turnover and consumption is an early and constant feature of the disease. Prostacyclin is a potent vasodilator and inhibitor of platelet aggregation and a deficiency of prostacyclin could account for these well documented features.

In pregnancy-associated hypertension the role of renin has been widely investigated. Many investigators set out to show that activation of the renin-angiotensin system played a part in the pathogenesis of pre-eclampsia but paradoxically found that the system is activated in normal pregnancy but suppressed in patients with pregnancy associated hypertension. Prostacyclin has been shown to promote renin secretion and prostacyclin deficiency could thus also explain the suppression of renin secretion in pre-eclampsia compared with the elevation seen in normal pregnancy (Miyamuri et al 1979). A relative deficiency of prostacyclin could also explain the increased sensitivity to angiotensin II observed in pregnancy associated hypertension compared with normal pregnancy (Lewis 1982, Remuzzi et al 1981).

Evidence of prostacyclin deficiency in pregnancies complicated by pre-eclampsia has now been demonstrated by several groups of workers. Patients with pre-eclampsia have less prostacyclin-like activity in amniotic fluid (Bodzenta et al 1980) and prostacyclin-like activity in uterine tissue from pre-eclamptic pregnancies yielded much lower levels than those obtained from normal pregnancies (Bussolino et al 1980). Several groups have shown, by differing methods, that umbilical arteries taken from fetuses associated with pre-eclamptic mothers contain less prostacyclin activity and less synthetic capability for production of prostacyclin compared with normal (Remuzzi et al 1980a, Downing et al 1982, Carrerras et al 1981).

Umbilical cords of infants born of pregnancies complicated by chronic placental insufficiency have been shown to produce less prostacyclin than cords obtained from infants born after normal pregnancy or acute placental insufficiency (Stuart et al 1981), suggesting that umbilical prostacyclin deficiency may be particularly associated with pre-eclampsia and intrauterine fetal growth retardation. *However the possibility that the reduced generation of PGI$_2$ by vascular tissue could be the consequence of the disease and not a primary cause cannot be excluded.* Much more experimental and clinical work will be necessary to clarify this problem (Carrerras et al 1981).

Platelets in pre-eclampsia

There have been many reports showing that the circulating platelet count is reduced in pre-eclampsia (Trudinger 1976, Howie 1977, Bonnar 1981). A significant inverse relation between platelet count and FDPs supports the concept that the fall in platelet count is due to increased consumption of platelets in DIC (Howie et al 1971). This decrease precedes any detectable rise in serum fibrin or fibrinogen degradation products in women subsequently developing pre-eclampsia according to Redman et al (1978). It has been suggested that platelet emboli are occurring in the microcirculation of the placenta which could be of special importance in relation to the diminished placental blood flow said to be a consistent finding in pre-eclampsia. The finding that circulating platelet levels of 5-hydroxytryptamine (5HT) are lower in pre-eclamptic pregnancy than during normal pregnancy and that the level is directly related to the severity of the condition (Howie 1977) lends support to this hypothesis. The explanation put forward is that after aggregation in the microcirculation and release of some of their 5HT the platelets then recirculate with reduced levels. Higher levels of 5-HT had been reported previously in the placenta of patients suffering from pre-eclampsia (Senior et al 1963). A further study (Whigham et al 1978) showed that with severe pre-eclampsia, in addition to reduced platelet levels of 5-HT, the platelets were less responsive to a variety of aggregating agents and that plasma adenine nucleotide levels were raised compared to those of normal pregnancy.

These findings could be explained by the platelets having undergone aggregation and disaggregation within the circulation, releasing active principles into the plasma in the process. A study of platelet lifespan during normal and pre-eclamptic pregnancy has shown that, although there is no difference between platelet lifespan in healthy nonpregnant and pregnant women, there is significant shortening of platelet survival during pregnancy complicated by pre-eclampsia (Rakoczi et al 1979).

Factor VIII in pre-eclampsia

During normal pregnancy the levels of both factor VIII-related antigens (factor VIIIRAg) and factor VIII coagulation activity (factor VIIIC) rise concomitantly (Whigham et al 1979, Fournie et al 1981).

An increased ratio between factor VIII related antigen and factor VIII coagulation activity (factor VIIIRAg:factor VIIIC increased) has been shown to be characteristic of pre-eclampsia (Redman et al 1977, Thornton & Bonnar 1977, Fournie et al 1981). Redman & colleagues (1977) showed that there was a high correlation between increasing factor VIIIRAg:factor VIIIC ratio and the severity of pre-eclampsia and Thornton & Bonnar (1977) showed a positive correlation between the increase in this ratio and both perinatal mortality and severe intrauterine fetal growth retardation. These

92

changes in factor VIII most likely indicate a low grade DIC and thrombin generation originating in the uteroplacental circulation (Bonnar & Sheppard 1981).

Soluble fibrin complexes in pre-eclampsia

Levels of soluble fibrin complexes are increased in patients with severe pre-ecalampsia (Howie et al 1971, McKillop et al 1976, Edgar et al 1977). During normal pregnancy a small amount of cryofibrinogen can be detected, but there is a more obvious increase in the level in women with pre-eclampsia (Howie et al 1971).

The majority of the soluble complexes are made up of fibrin-fibrinogen dimers (Edgar et al 1977). This would support the concept that the soluble complexes in pre-eclampsia result from low grade DIC, during the process of thrombin generation and the conversion of fibrinogen to fibrin (Bonnar & Sheppard 1981).

Fibrin degradation products in pre-ecalampsia

It is now an accepted fact that levels of FDPs during pregnancy complicated by pre-eclampsia are elevated above those found during normal pregnancy. Early studies (Bonnar et al 1971, Howie et al 1971) clearly demonstrated these increases and that the more severe the pathological process the greater the rise in FDPs — the highest levels being demonstrated in women during the 48 hours following an eclamptic seizure (Bonnar et al 1971). These findings were confirmed in a later study (Howie et al 1976). Urinary FDPs are not usually found during the course of normal pregnancy but are excreted in large quantities in patients with severe pre-eclampsia (Hedner & Astedt 1970). Postdelivery there is a further substantial increase in urinary FDPs (Howie et al 1971), still detectable six days after delivery (Condie & Ogston 1976).

Plasminogen activator in pre-eclampsia

The levels of fibrinolytic activator in the plasma are low during normal pregnancy and return to normal within one hour of delivery. The placenta has been shown to contain inhibitors of fibrinolysis and the fact that fibrinolytic activity is restored to normal following its delivery suggests that inhibition of fibrinolysis is mediated through this organ (Bonnar & Sheppard 1981). However the low levels of plasminogen activator could well be the result of absorption to fibrin which is normally laid down in the placental vessels and not due to active impaired fibrinolytic factors secreted by the placenta (Fletcher et al 1979). During pre-eclamptic pregnancy the plasminogen activator levels are even lower than during normal pregnancy and remain lower for three or more days following delivery (Bonnar et al 1971). This again supports the concept of DIC being part of the pathogenesis of pre-eclampsia, the low levels of plasminogen activity being the result of its increased activation in the removal of both intra- and extravascular fibrin (see below), the clearance of fibrin not being achieved until after delivery. This would also explain the continuing output of FDPs in the urine up to six days after delivery (see above).

Vascular deposition of fibrin in pre-eclampsia

The association of thrombus formation in the small vessels with eclampsia is by no means a recent discovery; many publications dating from 1893 (see Howie 1977) documented such lesions in fatal cases of eclampsia from histological examinations. There are technical difficulties, however, in demonstrating low-grade intra-vascular coagulation by histological methods and such postmortem studies cannot define the role of the haemostatic mechanisms in pre-eclampsia. The advent of electron-microscopy and improved methods of obtaining biopsy specimens from the placental bed and renal apparatus during life have allowed more meaningful studies of fibrin deposition during pregnancies complicated by hypertension, severe intrauterine fetal growth retardation or both (Howie 1977, Bonnar & Sheppard 1981).

There is general agreement that in pre-eclampsia there is a glomerular lesion which consists of swelling of the glomerular capillary endothelial cells and deposition of an amorphous fibroid material containing either fibrinogen or one of its derivatives (for references see Howie 1977). Biopsy specimens from the liver and the placental bed taken at caesarean section show similar deposition of fibrin and fibrinoid necrosis during pre-eclamptic pregnancies. Sheppard & Bonnar (1974) have shown fibrin and platelet deposition in the arterial supply of normal placentae using electron microscopy. This suggests that a mild compensated intravascular coagulation is a physiological process during normal pregnancy (see Ch. 1). In many subsequent studies they have shown that pre-eclamptic pregnancies, and particularly those associated with intrauterine fetal growth retardation, are associated with extensive atheromatous lesions with fibrin deposition and lipid-laden cells resulting in occlusion of some of the decidual spiral arteries of the placental bed.

Haematological management of pre-eclampsia

Although we still do not understand the pathogenesis of pre-eclampsia and eclampsia their management is more effective than it was 80 years ago when maternal mortality due to eclampsia occurred roughly once per hundred pregnancies. Eclampsia is now an uncommon endstage complication of undetected or mismanaged hypertension and maternal death is very rare.

In those women who do not respond to simple basic forms of management, the babies may suffer anything from mild IUGR to the extremes of succumbing in utero or failing to survive the neonatal period. Alternatively the hypertension is so completely out of control that the only way to prevent lifethreatening maternal eclampsia is to deliver the fetus whether or not it is viable. It is in women with these types of severe complications that attempts have been made to reduce the occlusive lesions in small vessels and thereby bring down the blood pressure as well as improve placental function. Howie & colleagues (1975) failed to affect the clinical course of three cases of severe pre-eclampsia using high-dose intravenous heparin together with the antiplatelet drug dipyridamole. However, given that the patient with severe pre-eclampsia or eclampsia is at risk of cerebral haemorrhage the use of heparin should be questioned. The introduction of small-dose subcutaneous heparin (Bonnar 1981) in the prophylaxis of venous thrombo-embolism soon led to the concept that, because of the association of low grade DIC with pre-eclampsia, this mode of delivering heparin might improve the outcome in hypertensive pregnancies. Unfortunately, while it proved possible to correct the platelet count and lower the FDPs as well as the factor VIIIRAg:factor VIIIC ratio in pre-eclampsic patients, there was no improvement in their fetal outcome.

Bonnar & Sheppard (1981) suggested that the likelihood of a successful pregnancy was improved where hypertension was well controlled and the patient treated with subcutaneous heparin and dipyridamole from the eighteenth week of gestation. However, if the activation of coagulation was mediated through the platelets in pre-eclampsia then very high levels of heparin would be required to inhibit platelet activation. A more logical approach would be to use antiplatelet agents to prevent or delay the onset of pre-eclampsia. Although I believe that several centres may be undertaking trials of antiplatelet agents, with or without small-dose heparin, in an attempt to prevent or ameliorate the course of pre-eclampsia, I have only been able to find one published report of such a study. Beaufils & colleagues (1982) in Paris conducted a prospective controlled study of dipyridamole and aspirin in high-risk pregnancy and reported preliminary results from 57 cases. The women were randomly allocated at three months gestation to the treatment group receiving dipyridamole 300 mg daily and low dose aspirin 150 mg/day, or the control group. There was a striking difference in the incidence of hypertension and fetal outcome in favour of the treated group. There were three fetal deaths in the control group and none in the treated group. In addition, antihypertensive drugs were required in 50% of the subjects in the treated group compared with 84% requiring antihypertensive therapy in the control group.

Current use of the antithrombotic drugs which act on platelets has been largely based on their ability to inhibit platelet cyclo-oxygenase, the foremost example being aspirin; this inhibits the generation of TX A_2 in platelets but can inhibit prostacyclin formation in the vessel wall too and therefore have a less beneficial effect (Moncada & Vane 1981). So far prostacyclin is the most potent and comprehensive inhibitor of all forms of aggregation. It has been used with relative therapeutic success in patients with Raynaud's syndrome (Belch et al 1983a) and in relieving pain in patients with severe occlusive arterial disease (Belch et al 1983b). Infusions of prostacyclin have also been tried in haemolytic uraemic syndrome in children and may have had a beneficial effect on the course of that disease (Beattie et al 1981, Webster et al 1980). One published report of an unsuccessful attempt to treat pregnancy associated hypertension and severe intrauterine growth retardation with infusion of prostacyclin at 25 weeks gestation led the authors to conclude that they started the administration of $PG1_2$ too late in the course of the disease (Lewis et al 1981).

The future of antithrombotic therapy in pre-eclampsia may well be in the development of compounds with a prostacyclin type of action but which are long-acting and orally effective.

Intrauterine fetal growth retardation

Pregnancies complicated by late fetal growth retardation show extensive atheromatous lesions with considerable fibrin deposition and accumulation of cells laden with lipid (Bonnar & Sheppard 1981). These changes are present whether the fetal growth retardation is associated with hypertension or not. It is likely that the abnormality in pre-eclampsia is a syndrome of disseminated intravascular coagulation but, during normotensive pregnancy complicated by intrauterine growth retardation, intravascular fibrin deposition is localised to the placenta. The factors responsible for the dissemination or localisation of the process are as yet unknown. Many of the ultrastructural characteristics in the uteroplacental arteries resemble those seen in human atheroma and atherosclerotic lesions of the coronary and cerebral arteries. They are also similar to the lesions seen in arteries in rejected renal transplants. Reduced maternal levels of circulating platelets have also been found to correlate with intrauterine growth retardation (Trudinger 1976).

Wallenburg & Rotmans (1982) have shown enhanced reactivity of the platelet thromboxane pathway in both normotensive and hypertensive pregnancy associated with impaired fetal growth. They suggested that the increased in vivo platelet activation and consumption in pregnancies with chronic placental insufficiency may be due to deficient placental vascular prostacyclin production.

It has recently been shown (Jogee et al 1983) that production of prostacyclin in vitro from human placental cells from pregnancies complicated by fetal growth retardation was significantly reduced compared with that in normal pregnancies. They suggest that defective $PG1_2$ production by cells of trophoblastic origin may be an important aetiological factor in the thrombotic occlusion of uteroplacental vessels, leading to impaired fetal growth.

So far, I know of no series of women at risk for impaired fetal growth being successfully managed using prostacyclin infusions from early pregnancy, although this is an obvious area for investigation. Again, as in the treatment for pre-eclampsia, the future must be in the development of drugs with a prostacyclin-like activity which are long acting and orally effective (De Gaetano et al 1982).

REFERENCES

Bamford D S, Jogee M, Williams K I 1980 Prostacyclin formation by the pregnant human myometrium. British Journal of Obstetrics and Gynaecology 87: 215–218

Beattie T J, Murphy A V, Willoughby M L N, Belch J J F 1981 Prostacyclin infusion in haemolytic uraemia syndrome of children. British Medical Journal 283: 470

Beaufils M, Uzan S, Donsimoni R, Colau J C 1982 A prospective controlled study of Dipyridamole and aspirin in high risk pregnancy. Preliminary results in 57 cases. Clinical and Experimental Hypertension Bl: 334

Belch et al 1983a Intermittent epoprostenol (prostacyclin) infusion in patients with Raynaud's syndrome, Lancet i: 313–315

Belch et al 1983b Epoprostenol (prostacyclin) and severe arterial disease. A double blind trial. Lancet i: 315–317

Bodzenta A, Thomson J M, Poller L (1980) Prostacyclin activity in amniotic fluid in pre-eclampsia. Lancet ii: 650

Bonnar J 1976 Coagulation disorders. Journal of Clinical Pathology 29: (suppl. 10) 35–41

Bonnar J (1981) Haemostasis and coagulation disorders in pregnancy. In: Bloom A L, Thomas P P (eds) Haemostasis and thrombosis, Churchill Livingstone, Edinburgh p 454–471

Bonnar J, McNicol G P, Douglas A S 1971 Coagulation and fibrinolytic systems in pre-eclampsia and eclampsia British Medical Journal ii: 12–16

Bonnar J, Sheppard B L 1981 Coagulation activation and local vascular changes in pre-eclampsia. In: Brod J (ed) Kidney and pregnancy contributions to nephrology 25. Karger, Basel, p 98–107

Bussolino F, Benedetto C, Massobrio M, Camussi G 1980 Maternal vascular prostacylcin activity in pre-eclampsia. Lancet ii: 702

Carreras L O, De Freyn G, Van Houtte E, Vermylen J, Van Assche A 1981 Prostacyclin and pre-eclampsia. Lancet i: 442

Condie R G, Ogston D 1976, Sequential studies on components of the haemostatic mechanism in pregnancy with particular reference to the development of pre-eclampsia. Journal of Obstetrics and Gynaecology of the British Commonwealth 83: 938–942

Downing I, Shepherd G L, Lewis P J 1982 Kinetics of prostacyclin synthetase in umbilical artery microsomes from normal and pre-eclamptic pregnancies. British Journal of Clinical Pharmacology 13: 195–198

Edgar W, McKillop C, Howie P W 1977 Composition of soluble fibrin complexes in pre-eclampsia. Thrombosis Research 10: 567–574

Fletcher A P, Alkjaersig N K, Burstein R 1979, The influence of pregnancy upon blood coagulation and plasma fibrinolytic enzyme function. American Journal of Obstetrics and Gynecology 134: 743–751

Fournie A, Monrozies M, Pontonnier G, Boneu B, Bierne R 1981 Factor VIII complex in normal pregnancy, pre-eclampsia and fetal growth retardation. British Journal of Obstetrics and Gynaecology 88: 250–254

De Gaetano G, Cerletti C, Bertele V 1982 Pharmacology of antiplatelet drugs and clinical trials on thrombosis prevention: a difficult link. Lancet ii: 974–977

Hedner U, Astedt B 1970 Fibrinolytic split products in serum and urine in pregnancy. Acta obstetrica gynaecologica scandinavica 49: 363–366

Howie P W 1977 The haemostatic mechanisms in pre-eclampsia. Clinics in Obstetrics and Gynaecology 4: 595–611

Howie P W 1979 Blood clotting and fibrinolysis in pregnancy. Postgraduate Medical Journal 55: 362–366

Howie P W, Prentice C R M, Forbes C D 1975 Failure of heparin therapy to affect the clinical course of severe pre-eclampsia. British Journal of Obstetrics and Gynaecology 82: 711–717

Howie P W, Prentice C R M, McNicol G P 1971 Coagulation fibrinolysis and platelet function in pre-eclampsia, essential hypertension and placental insufficiency. Journal of Obstetrics and Gynaecology of the British Commonwealth 78: 992–1003

Howie P W, Purdie D W, Begg C B, Prentice C R M 1970 Use of coagulation tests to predict the clinical progress of pre-eclampsia. Lancet ii: 323–325

Jogee M, Myatt L, Elder M G 1983 Decreased prostacyclin production by placental cells in culture from pregnancies complicated by fetal growth retardation. British Journal of Obstetrics and Gynaecology 90: 247–250

Lewis P J 1982 The role of prostacyclin in pre-eclampsia. British Journal of Hospital Medicine 28: 393–395

Lewis P J and Boylan P 1979 Fetal breathing: a review. American Journal of Obstetrics and Gynecology 134: 587–598

Lewis P J, Boylan P, Friedman L A, Hensby C N, Downing I 1980 Prostacyclin in pregnancy. British Medical Journal i: 1581–1582

Lewis P J et al 1981 Prostacyclin and pre-eclampsia. Lancet i: 559

McKay D G 1981 Chronic intravascular coagulation in normal pregnancy and pre-eclampsia. Contributions to Nephrology 25: 108–119

McKillop C, Howie P W, Forbes C D 1976 Soluble fibrinogen-fibrin complexes in pre-eclampsia. Lancet i: 56–58

MacGillivray I 1981 Raised blood pressure in pregnancy. Aetiology of pre-eclampsia. British Journal of Hospital Medicine 26: 110–119

Mäkilä U-M, Jouppila P, Kirkinen P, Viinikka L, Vlikorkala O 1983 Relation between umbilical prostacyclin production and blood flow in the fetus. Lancet i: 728–729

Mitchell M D, Keirse M J N C, Brunt J D, Andersen A B M, Turnbull A C 1979 Concentration of the prostacyclin metabolite 6-keto prostaglandin F_1 alpha in amniotic fluid during late pregnancy and labour. British Journal of Obstetrics and Gynaecology 86: 350–353

Miyamuri I, Fitzgerald G A, Brown M J, Lewis P J 1979 Prostacyclin stimulates the renin-angiotensin aldosterone system in man. Journal of Clinical. Endocrinology and Metabolism 49: 943–944

Moncada M D, Vane J R 1979 Arachidonic acid metabolites and the interactions between platelets and blood-vessel walls. The New England Journal of Medicine 300: 1142–1147

Moncada S, Vane J R 1981 Prostacyclin: normostatic regulator or biological curiosity? Clinical Science 61: 369–392

Myatt L, Elder M G 1977 Inhibition of platelet aggregation by a placental substance with prostacyclin-like activity. Nature 268: 159–160

O'Grady J, Moody S G 1982 Prostaglandins, platelets and vascular disease. Hospital Update 8: 1475–1486

Rakoczi T, Tallian F, Bagdany S, Gati I 1979 Platelet lifespan in normal pregnancy and pre-eclampsia as determined by a nonradioisotope technique. Thrombosis Research 15: 553–556

Redman C W G 1979 Coagulation problems in human pregnancy. Postgraduate Medical Journal 55: 367–371

Redman C W G, Bonnar J, Bellin C 1978 Early platelet consumption in pre-eclampsia. British Medical Journal 1: 467–469

Redman C W G, Brennecke S P, Mitchell M D 1981 Prostaglandins and pre-eclampsia. Lancet i: 731

Redman C W G, Denson K W E, Beilin L J, Bolton F G, Stirrat G M 1977 Factor VIII consumption in pre-eclampsia. Lancet ii: 1249–1259

Remuzzi G, et al 1978 Haemolytic ureamia syndrome: deficiency of plasma factor(s) regulating prostacyclin activity. Lancet ii: 871–872

Remuzzi G et al 1979 Prostacyclin and human foetal circulation. Prostaglandins 18: 341–348

Remuzzi et al 1980a Reduction of fetal vascular prostacyclin activity in pre-eclampsia. Lancet ii: 310

Remuzzi G et al 1980b Prostacyclin generation by cultured endothelial cells in haemolytic uraemic syndrome. Lancet i: 656–657

Remuzzi G et al 1981 Plasmatic regulation of vascular prostacyclin in pregnancy. British Medical Journal 282: 512–514

Ritter J M, Barrow S E, Blair I A, Dollery C T 1983 Release of prostacyclin in vivo and its role in man. Lancet i: 317–319

Senior J B, Fahim I, Sullivan F M, Robson J M 1983 Possible role of 5-hydroxytryptamine in toxaemia of pregnancy. Lancet ii: 553–554

Sheppard B L, Bonnar J 1974 The ultrastructure of the arterial supply of the human placenta in early and late pregnancy. Journal of Obstetrics and Gynaecology of the British Commonwealth 81: 497–511

Stuart M J et al 1981 Decreased prostacyclin production: a characteristic of chronic placental insufficiency syndromes. Lancet i: 1126–1128

Thornton C A, Bonnar J 1977 Factor VIII-related antigen and factor VIII coagulant activity in normal and pre-eclamptic pregnancy. Journal of Obstetrics and Gynaecology of the British Commonwealth 81: 497–511

Trudinger B J 1976 Platelets and intrauterine growth retardation in pre-eclampsia. British Journal of Obstetrics and Gynaecology 83: 284–286

Wallenburg H C S, Rotmans N 1982 Enhanced reactivity of the platelet thromboxane pathway in normotensive and hypertensive pregnancies with insufficient fetal growth. American Journal of Obstetrics and Gynecology 144: 523–528

Webster J 1983 Antiplatelet drugs. British Journal of Hospital Medicine 30: 45–50

Webster J, Rees A J, Lewis J P, Hensby C N 1980 Prostacyclin deficiency in haemolytic ureamia syndrome. British Medical Journal 281: 271

Whigham K A E, Howie P W, Drummond A H, Prentice C R M 1978 Abnormal platelet function in pre-eclampsia. British Journal of Obstetrics and Gynaecology 85: 28–32

Whigham K A E, Howie P W, Shah M M, Prentice C R M 1979 Factor VIII-related antigen and coagulant activity in intrauterine growth retardation. Thrombosis Research 16: 629–638

Whigham K A E, Howie P W, Shah M M, Prentice C R M 1980 Factor VIII related antigen/coagulant activity ratio as a predictor of fetal growth retardation: A comparison with hormone and uric acid measurements. British Journal of Obstetrics and Gynaecology 87: 797–803

5

Acquired defects of haemostasis during pregnancy

Immune thrombocytopenic purpura

A low pregnancy platelet count is most frequently associated with DIC as already described. Sometimes severe megaloblastic anaemia of pregnancy is accompanied by thrombocytopenia but the platelet count rapidly returns to normal after therapy with folic acid (Bonnar 1981).

Toxic depression of bone marrow megakaryocytes during pregnancy can occur in association with infection, certain drugs and alcoholism; neoplastic infiltration may also result in thrombo-cytopenia. Probably the single most important cause of isolated thrombocytopenia is immune thrombocytopenia purpura (ITP) which is a disease primarily of young women in their reproductive years (McMillan 1981). The diagnosis used to be made when severe thrombocytopenia was found to be associated with normal or increased numbers of megakaryocytes in the bone marrow but there are now more reliable tests for demonstrating the responsible IgG antibody (Van Leeuwen et al 1981, Hegde et al 1981). This antibody is directed against and coats the platelet which is rapidly removed from the circulation by the reticulo-endothelial system. It is now possible to distinguish between IgG antibodies which can cross the placenta and IgM antibodies which cannot (Van Leeuwen et al 1981) as well as identifying platelet-bound antibody and the more dangerous free IgG antibody in the maternal plasma (Hegde et al 1981). Much of the published literature (Carloss et al 1980, Territo et al 1973, Terao et al 1981) consists of retrospective analyses of women suffering from ITP managed throughout pregnancy without the advantage of these new, more reliable tests which identify platelet autoantibodies.

The maternal platelet count should be checked regularly during pregnancy and if it falls below $20 \times 10^9/l$ then steroids are indicated. These should be tapered to the lowest dose that provides safe platelet counts (McMillan 1981, Carloss et al 1980) because eclampsia, hypertension and psychosis are not unusual in addition to the common side effects. Adrenal suppression may adversely affect fetal development and therefore the use of steroids should be reserved for those cases where the ITP is thought to be a serious risk to the mother (Carloss et al 1980).

Splenectomy during pregnancy should probably be avoided because there appears to be an appreciable maternal mortality rate which does not exist in nonpregnant women (Bell 1977). However, this information was collected from cases operated on before the advent of modern supportive therapy and might not be applicable to modern-day practice.

Because the IgG antibody will cross the placenta it will reduce the fetal count too and the major risk is that of intracranial bleeding during delivery. If there is any question that a vaginal delivery will be hazardous then elective caesarean section should be undertaken though assessing this poses a considerable clinical dilemma. It has been recommended by several authors (see Carloss et al 1980) that if the maternal platelet count is less than $100 \times 10^9/l$, indicating active ITP, then caesarean section should be performed. However, risks to the mother must be balanced against risks to the fetus, particularly when the fetal platelet count cannot be determined. A recent study of 41 pregnancies in 38 patients with ITP from Canada (Kelton et al 1982) showed that the maternal platelet count was not related to the platelet count in the fetus but that maternal platelet associated antibody was predictive of infant platelet count. McMillan (1981) states that caesarean section is indicated if the maternal spleen is absent regardless of platelet count. If, however, one has access to reliable and reproducible platelet antibody tests and no appreciable platelet-bound or free maternal autoantibody can be demonstrated, this may not be necessary.

If an easy vaginal delivery is expected in a term baby this should present no more risk of intracranial bleeding than a caesarean section. It should be remembered that a caesarean section in the presence of maternal thrombocytopenia carries considerable risk of haemorrhage from the incisions (not from the placental site which is protected by normal myometrial contraction). Although transfused platelets will have a short life in the maternal circulation due to the antibody, they will help to achieve haemostasis of the wound and should be given to the mother at delivery.

A method for direct measurement of the fetal platelet count in scalp blood obtained transcervically prior to or early in labour, has recently been described (Ayromlooi 1978, Scott et al 1980). The authors recommend that caesarean section should be performed in all cases where the fetal platelet count is less than $50 \times 10^9/l$. This approach is more logical than a decision concerned with the mode of delivery based on the maternal platelet count and splenectomy status, but is not without risk to the fetus from haemorrhage if the count is low. If reliable platelet antibody tests are available and have been performed throughout the antenatal period the decision concerning the necessity for caesarean section and its timing can be taken at leisure, based on a rational assessment of disease activity and the risk to the mother and fetus. Chronic ITP as opposed to acute ITP is the usual clinical form in adults. It remains refractory to all forms of conventional treatment in 30% of cases (Difino et al 1980).

A chance observation that two children with agammaglobulinanaemia and thrombocytopenia treated with intravenous IgG had recovery of their platelet count to normal levels led to further studies in children with ITP (Imbach et al 1981). All responded with increased platelet count but in children the spontaneous remission rate is high and it is difficult to judge the true efficacy of intravenous IgG if used in such acute forms of the disease. Newland & colleagues (1983) have recently published the effect of this form of treatment in 25 adults with acute and chronic forms of ITP. All responded with an increase in the platelet count above pretreatment levels. There was no difference between splenectomised and nonsplenectomised individuals, whether over or under 40 years of age, or whose history was longer or shorter than one year. It is known that intravenous administration of monomeric polyvalent human IgG in doses greater than that produced endogenously prolongs the clearance time of immune particles by the reticulo-endothelial systems (RES). It is thus thought that in ITP such a prolongation of clearance of IgG coated platelets by the RES results in an increase in the number of circulating platelets, but the mechanism is as yet unknown. It has been suggested (Salama et al 1981) that after infusion of high doses of IgG red cells become coated and as they far outnumber the other cellular elements of the blood they will be preferentially sequestered in the RES. The macrophages will rapidly become saturated by coated red cells even if only a small number are involved, leaving platelets (and neutrophils) free in the circulation. This hypothesis would explain the fact that immunoglobulin therapy is ineffective in the treatment of autoimmune haemolytic anaemia and that platelet counts rise in some ITP patients after induction of a mild haemolytic syndrome by injection of anti-Rh$_o$(D) (Salama et al 1983).

At the time of writing I can find only two reports of the use of this therapy for ITP in pregnancy with successful outcome. A single case reported from the United Kingdom (Morgenstern et al 1983) highlighted the efficacy of high dose intravenous IgG in chronic ITP which had failed to respond to steroids. A primigravida who presented in the 11th week of pregnancy with thrombocytopenia of 16 years duration had persistently low platelet counts (around 10×10^9/l) and recurrent epistaxes throughout the antenatal period. After 7 weeks of prednisolone 40 mg daily the platelet count remained dangerously low at 7×10^9/l. Accordingly in the 38th week of pregnancy an IgG infusion (Sandoglobulin) was started at a dose of 0.4 g/kg/day for 5 days according to the manufacturer's instructions. On the fifth day of infusion the membranes ruptured spontaneously and delivery of a normal baby girl, whose platelet count was 253×10^9/l, followed 28 hours later. The maternal platelet count at delivery was only 25×10^9/l but had risen to 175×10^9/l by the following day.

The authors recommend that infusion of IgG should be started 10–15 days before the expected date of delivery to allow sufficient time for maximal response to the infusion. Peak platelet counts are usually reached 4 days after the end of the infusion. *High dose immunoglobulin crosses the placenta and should therefore ensure normal platelet counts in both mother and fetus, whatever the mechanism of action.*

Wenske & colleagues (1983) reported two pregnant women with severe ITP during late pregnancy. In both cases a rising platelet count response was obtained five days after induction of high dose immunoglobulin therapy but a second course was required to obtain a safe maternal platelet count for delivery. The authors made the point that varying amount of IgG may be necessary to produce blockade of RES and increase the platelet count in individual patients. They also draw attention to the high costs of IgG therapy which may have limited its use so far in the routine treatment of ITP. The cheaper alternative of long-term steroid therapy may have adverse effects on both mother and fetus and as IgG therapy has no expected side effects it is an effective and perhaps preferable alternative treatment. Even without the introduction of more recent aids to diagnosis of activity of the disease and treatment with high dose IgG, the maternal death rate has fallen from 8–9 per cent in 1950 to virtually zero. The outlook for the fetus, which previously had a death rate of about 26% is also much improved (Epstein et al 1950, Terao et al 1981).

Alloimmune thrombocytopenia

In a situation in which fetal platelets carry antigens not present on the maternal platelets, antibodies may be produced by the mother against these fetal cells (cf. Rh.D haemolytic disease of the newborn). It has been established that isoimmune or alloimmune neonatal thrombocytopenia occurs about 1 in 10 000 births. Although not strictly a haemostatic problem of pregnancy in that the mother is at no risk, the situation is very similar to that in which the mother has ITP with IgG platelet-associated immune antibody but a normal platelet count (e.g. postsplenectomy) and the hazard for the fetus is exactly the same. The management of delivery in identified cases at risk is as described above. I have included this rare problem of thrombocytopenia in the fetus with the more frequent complications of ITP in the mother because the two conditions are often confused (Kelton et al 1980).

Paternally derived platelet antigens stimulating maternal antibody formation may be restricted to the platelets but some are shared with white cells and may be identical with antigens of the HL-A system. The platelet antigen most commonly associated with isoimmune neonatal thrombocytopenia has been designated Pl^{A1} (also known as Zw^a). It is confined to the platelet and is responsible for more than 50% of proven cases of isoimmune neonatal purpura. In population surveys 98% of individuals prove to be Pl^{A1} (Zw^a) positive. It is the 2% of women who are Pl^{A1} (Zw^a) negative who may give birth to an affected infant. The incidence is low, 1–2 per 10 000, but neonatal deaths due mainly to intracranial haemorrhage have occurred in 14% of documented cases. The diagnosis of isoimmune purpura depends on the combination of congenital thrombocytopenia, normal maternal platelet count, negative history of ITP and no evidence in the infant of any systemic disease such as infection or malignancy.

Screening for alloimmune neonatal purpura

It is not practical or possible to anticipate the first case of isoimmune purpura in a particular family but once a case has occurred it is valuable to obtain platelet genotypes of the parents. If the father is homozygous Pl^{Al} (Zw^a) positive and the mother a sensitised Pl^{Al} (Zw^a) negative, all subsequent infants are likely to be affected. The IgG platelet antibody, free in the mother's serum, can be identified (Hegde et al 1981). Corticosteriod therapy to the mother immediately before delivery is recommended because of the nonspecific affect it has which may protect the fetus from haemorrhage in the face of thrombocytopenia. Elective atraumatic delivery with a strong consideration of caesarean section is indicated. Washed maternal platelet concentrates or Pl^{Al} (Zw^a) negative platelets should be available for administration to the infant immediately after birth. All infants of a mother with a previous history of this disorder should be screened for neonatal thrombocytopenia.

If the Pl^{Al}(Zw^a) antigen is not involved in a family thought to be at risk for isoimmune purpura, an effort should be made to demonstrate an antibody in the maternal circulation directed against the father's platelets. Management of the subsequent pregnancy is as above with particular emphasis on atraumatic delivery. Washed maternal platelets should be used to treat any bleeding. Exchange transfusion will wash out the maternal antibody in the infant's circulation.

Whether infusion of high dose IgG to the mother before delivery has a place in the management of isoimmune neonatal thrombocytopenia has yet to be established, but its administration should theoretically result in an increased fetal platelet count.

Thrombotic thrombocyptopenic purpura

Thrombotic thrombocytopenic purpura (TTP) and haemolytic, uraemic syndrome (HUS) are two conditions associated with acute severe damage to small blood vessels, microangiopathic haemolytic anaemia, thrombocytopenia, renal failure and fluctuating neuro-logical signs. Clinically and pathologically TTP and HUS merge into one entity (Ingram et al 1982). A common basis for these two diseases has been suggested by the description of TTP and HUS in HLA identical siblings (Hellman et al 1980). The main differences are the more generalised manifestation of TTP and the localised renal damage in HUS and the age of the patients.

TTP is a disorder of young adults, predominantly women. The most common presenting features are fever, haemorrhages into skin and mucous membrane, oliguria or anuria and fits, hemiparesis and altered consciousness. The disease is usually rapidly progressive and fatal. HUS is predominantly a disorder of infants and young children who present with acute intravascular haemolysis and renal failure, often preceded by a short febrile illness, commonly gastro-enteritis. Several hundred patients with each condition have been reported but among these there have been only approximately 30 cases of women in pregnancy with TTP (Atlas et al 1982, May et al 1976). Both conditions are of unknown aetiology but an essential requisite of the pathogenesis is damage to the wall of small vessels. There is no doubt that local intravascular coagulation contributes to the vascular damage. In HUS the hyaline material laid down on basement membranes and occluding glomerular arterioles is rich in fibrin and in TTP the occluding material in arterioles and capillaries is also rich in fibrin, but laboratory and clinical evidence of DIC has only rarely been documented in association with this condition (Ingram et al 1982, Atlas et al 1982). It has been shown that plasminogen activator is absent from the wall of occluded vessels in TTP (Kwaan et al 1968) but whether this is primary or secondary is not clear. There is heightened platelet aggregability and plasma from patients with the problem induces platelet aggregation of platelets from normal donors (Lian et al 1979). It has been suggested therefore that the plasma of patients with TTP lacks an inhibitor which allows intravascular platelet aggregation leading to widespread micro-vascular damage. Remission can be induced and the defect corrected by administration of fresh frozen plasma (Lian et al 1979). It has been suggested by several groups that the missing inhibitor of platelet aggregation in TTP stimulates the production of PGI_2. Circulating PGI_2 levels were low in all four cases studied by Maclean & colleagues (1981) and in a further two cases from Italy prostacyclin synthesis stimulating factors were found to be low (Stratta et al 1983). Some patients fail to remit on simple plasma infusions but respond after plasmapheresis or after exchange transfusion and it has been suggested that soluble immune complexes are responsible for vascular damage leading to organ dysfunction.

Because HUS and TTP are sometimes associated with systemic lupus erythematosus and related disorders it has been suggested that the reticulo-endothelial system (RES) may have an important role to play. The capacity of the RES to clear potentially damaging substances such as immune complexes, SFMC, platelet micro-aggregates etc., is greatly reduced during the course of such conditions (Ingram et al 1982).

Possibly the most crucial problem when dealing with TTP is to establish a correct diagnosis (Atlas et al 1982). The condition can be confused with severe pre-eclampsia and placentae abruptio, especially if DIC is triggered also, although evidence of DIC is not often associated with TTP. ITP is another important condition to consider when confronted with a low platelet count. It is important to identify the platelet IgG antibody which is invariably present with active ITP and to remember that the fetus is *not* at risk for thrombocyptopenia in TTP, presumably because the postulated plasma factor involved in the pathogenesis does not cross the placenta.

The management of TTP remains difficult and not always successful since the aetiology and pathogenesis are poorly understood. But once the correct diagnosis has been made the management of TTP in principle is the same whether the patient is pregnant or not. The fetus is involved only in as far as it may suffer from placental insufficiency but it is not directly involved in the disease process. The logical approach is to give fresh frozen plasma as a source of the missing inhibitory factor and an antiplatelet agent which will not interfere with prostacyclin production such as dipyridamole or low dose aspirin to reduce platelet aggregability (Ingram et al 1982). If these measures fail, infusions of PGI_2 or plasmapheresis and exchange transfusion may be tried. If all these measures fail steroids, immunosuppressants and splenectomy are usually tried but their value is not clear from the few reports in the literature (Ingram et al 1982, Atlas et al 1982).

Atlas & colleagues (1982) successfully treated a primigravida with intrauterine fetal death at 20 weeks using repeated plasmapheresis.

Fresh frozen plasma and dipyridamole were used to treat two pregnant women in Italy (Stratta et al 1983); in both cases, although the women made a full recovery, the fetus was lost. This prompted the authors to speculate that some form of endothelial injury, damaging the fetoplacental microvasculature and leading to haemolysis and thrombocytopenia could result in the 'haemolytic abortion syndrome' and be responsible for recurrent unexplained miscarriages. The similarity between TTP and HUS might be of great importance in the light of the successful management of haemolytic uraemic syndrome in pregnancy using prostacyclin infusions (Webster et al 1980).

Systematic lupus erythematosus (SLE)

Systemic lupus erythematosus (SLE) is an autoimmune disorder which has a high incidence in women of childbearing years. It is a multisystem disorder with clinical manifestations which include skin rashes, arthritis, nephritis, disorders of the central nervous system (c.n.s.), haemolytic anaemia, thrombocytopenia and coagulation abnormalities. An essential finding for its accurate diagnosis is evidence of an antibody directed against nuclear material (antinuclear antibody — ANA). The condition is not rare compared with that of, say, TTP.

A recent report (Lubbe et al 1983) described the course and outcome of pregnancy in 10 women with SLE collected over 3 years in a hospital that delivers 5000 women per year; investigation was confined to women with overt clinical manifestations. The course was unpredictable but patients with mild disease seemed to have a better prognosis than those presenting with active c.n.s., renal or serosal disease.

The management of SLE during pregnancy does not differ substantially from that of the nonpregnant patient. The risk of steroid complications, particularly infection during pregnancy is less than the morbidity and fetal loss rate associated with an exacerbation of the underlying disease (Varner et al 1983). It is unwise to discontinue azothioprine therapy or reduce steroid dosage during gestation (Fine et al 1981). Appropriate steroid administration should be instituted or continued throughout pregnancy and the puerperium as needed to control clinical manifestations of the disease. Immunosuppressive drugs are considered teratogenic but the effect must be relatively weak or infrequent in view of the growing number of patients, such as those with a renal transplant, treated with them throughout pregnancy, yet having normal infants. It has been suggested that immunosuppressed women give birth to small-for-gestational-age infants with greater than expected frequency (Pitkin 1980), but more data are needed.

Thrombocytopenia and SLE

SLE is frequently complicated by thrombocytopenia but this is seldom severe, less than 5% of cases having platelet counts below $30 \times 10^9/l$ during the course of the disease (Hughes 1979). Thrombocytopenia is often the first presenting feature and may antedate any other manifestation of the disease by months or even years. Such patients are often labelled as suffering from ITP. Platelet associated IgG is often found on testing (Hegde et al 1977) but it is not clear whether the positive result is due to antiplatelet antibody, immune complexes or both. The management of thrombocytopenia associated with SLE in pregnancy does not differ substantially from that of ITP, but immunosuppressive therapy should not be diminished or discontinued during pregnancy (Varner et al 1983). Carefully monitored doses of corticosteroids and azothiaprine are invaluable in controlling all manifestations of the disease.

Circulating anticoagulants associated with systemic lupus erythematosus

Inactivators directed against specific clotting factors, particularly factor VIII, may arise in patients with SLE and will be discussed below. The most frequent 'lupus anticoagulant' of the various types which may develop in SLE is present in 5–10% of all patients (Ingram et al 1982). It inhibits the interaction between the prothrombin activator (complex of factor Xa, factor V, phospholipid and calcium) and prothrombin but the precise mode of action is not known. Phospholipid is the likely site of inhibition because other abnormalities involving phospholipid are found in systemic lupus. False positive tests for syphilis, for example, are common; the cardiolipin antigen for this test is derived from ox-heart phospholipid. Most anticoagulants studied immunochemically turn out to be IgG but some are IgM or mixtures of both.

The diagnosis is based on finding a prolonged partial thromboplastin time which is not corrected by normal plasma. This anticoagulant was originally described in patients suffering from SLE hence the term 'lupus anticoagulant' but it is not confined to such patients and may occur in other diseases, particularly haematological malignant conditions. In one analysis (Boxer et al 1976) SLE was found in 40% of patients with circulating lupus anticoagulant but only 5% of patients who satisfied the diagnostic criteria for SLE were found to have that specific anticoagulant. The lupus anticoagulant can occur in patients without any symptoms, signs or serological evidence of SLE apart from a positive antinuclear antibody test (Lubbe et al 1983).

Bleeding is a rare clinical manifestation unless a second haemostatic defect such as thrombocytopenia is also present. Patients do not bleed excessively even when undergoing major surgery; indeed, somewhat paradoxically, some patients experience thrombotic complications (Mueh et al 1980, Boey et al 1983, Hughes 1983).

The cause of the increased risk of thrombosis in patients with the lupus anticoagulant has yet to be determined though in some patients with SLE a lowered threshold for platelet aggregation induced by arachidonic acid has been shown (Marchesi et al 1981). Suppression of prostacyclin formation in vessel walls may play a part (Carreras et al 1981). In pregnancy the clinical outcome of the presence of the lupus anticoagulant extends further than its association with thrombosis. It is likely that this maternal thrombotic tendency compromises the blood supply to the placenta by causing extensive coagulation necrosis and intravillous thrombosis. Placental thrombosis and infarction lead to a high incidence of intrauterine death (Nilsson et al 1975, Carreras et al 1981, Lubbe et al 1983).

Without therapy the lupus anticoagulant persists for many years, whereas administration of steroids in the treatment of SLE often results in its reduction or disappearance. This has special significance for the management of SLE in pregnancy, illustrated by a recent study of 10 pregnant women with an identified circulating lupus anticoagulant (Lubbe et al 1983). Twenty-eight pregnancies occurred in the 10 women before treatment, 25 of which terminated unsuccessfully. Seven of these 10 women were treated during the course of a subsequent pregnancy with immunosuppressive doses of prednisone 40–60 mg per day and with aspirin 75 mg per day, to counteract the low threshold for platelet aggregation. The aim of the therapy was to establish whether live babies could be obtained if the abnormal complication was corrected. The prolonged in vitro PTT was brought back into the normal range in 5 pregnancies and live-births occurred in all 5 women; an abortion at 16 weeks gestation occurred in a woman in whom the PTT had not been reduced to the normal range.

The unrecognised presence of the LE anticoagulant may explain the high rate of fetal loss in women with SLE (Grigor et al 1977, Hughes 1983). In view of the successful outcome of pregnancies in women in whom the lupus anticoagulant had been suppressed Lubbe & colleagues (1983) recommend that the presence of this anticoagulant should be excluded in all women at risk. As soon as the LE anticoagulant is identified in pregnancy prednisone 40 mg per day should be started and if reduction in the clotting time is not achieved after 2 weeks the dose should be increased to 60 mg per day. The dose of aspirin at 75 mg per day, is only equivalent to one paediatric tablet and there were no haemorrhagic problems with this small dose. This is not surprising when it is realised that the haemostatic problems described in both mother and neonate by Stuart and colleagues

(1982) were associated with a maternal intake of 5–15 g daily during the 2 weeks prior to delivery.

The fact that the suppression of maternal lupus anticoagulant can be achieved safely and that this is associated with a dramatic reduction in the high fetal loss rate offers great hope for future pregnancies in women with such an anticoagulant.

Systemic lupus erythematosus in liveborn infants

Haemolytic anaemia, leukopenia and thrombocytopenia have all been observed in infants of women with active disease, presumably due to IgG antibody involved in the disease process crossing the placenta. But by no means all infants with passively acquired LE antibody demonstrate haematological abnormalities though the reasons for these discrepancies are not clear. LE cells have been demonstrated in the infant for up to 7 weeks postdelivery and antinuclear antibody has been shown to persist for as long as 15 weeks. If the passage of antibody results in haemolytic anaemia, thrombocytopenia or leukopenia, responses to steroids can be expected, and the transmitted disease process is transient (c.f. Rh haemolytic disease, ITP).

It would seem sensible to screen cord blood of all newborn infants of mothers suffering from SLE for the presence of LE factor, together with a full blood count, platelet count and direct antiglobulin (Coombs) test so that problems of management in the neonatal period can be anticipated.

Factor VIII antibody

An inhibitor of antihaemophilic factor is a rare cause of haemorrhage in previously healthy postpartum women (O'Brien 1954, Marengo-Rowe et al 1972, Voke & Letsky 1976, Coller et al 1981, Reece et al 1982). There are less than 50 documented cases in the literature (Voke & Letsky 1977, Reece et al 1982). Women who may have had this type of haemorrhagic disorder were first reported in the late 1930s and the nature of the defect was first reported in 1946 when the plasma of two such patients was shown not only to resemble haemophilic plasma but to have an inhibitory effect on normal clotting. In the late 1960s it was demonstrated that these inhibitors of factor VIII were immunoglobulins, as are the factor VIII antibodies found in treated haemophiliacs (for references see Voke & Letsky 1977). Of the postpartum coagulation defects of this type reported nearly all were found to be directed against factor VIII on in vitro testing. Only two were found to be antifactor IX antibodies.

Aetiology

The aetiology of antibodies to factor VIII is complex. The appearance of anti-VIIIC in nonhaemophilic individuals is usually attributed to an autoimmune process, or to isoimmunisation in women postpartum (Ingram et al 1982). However, no difference between maternal and fetal factor VIII has been demonstrated and neutralisation of both maternal and fetal factor VIII by the antibody is similar. There is at present no definite experimental evidence that factor VIII antigen allotypes exist. If the bleeding tendency is to be explained the antibody formed by stimulation of the maternal immune system by fetal factor VIII has to crossreact with maternal factor VIII. One would expect such an antibody to reappear after some of the subsequent pregnancies (cf. Rhesus sensitisation) but relapses have not been reported. Assuming that these inhibitors are IgG antibodies they are likely to cross the placenta and persist for several weeks in the neonate as do anti-Rhesus or antiviral antibodies. However, although factor VIII antibody and low levels of factor VIIIC have been found in the neonate born to mothers with antibody there have been no case reports of haemorrhagic problems in their offspring. The variable nature of this disorder argues in favour of a more complex pathogenesis. There is an association between factor VIII antibodies and autoimmune disorders such as rheumatoid arthritis and systemic lupus. There is also a well-known alteration of immune reactivity in normal pregnancy. These two observations suggest that a likely explanation of postpartum factor VIII antibodies is a temporary breakdown in mother's tolerance to her own factor VIII (or factor IX). This rare disorder does resemble other autoimmune states: its variable onset and duration; its varying severity; and in the fact that its aetiology is still a mystery (Voke & Letsky 1977).

Clinical manifestations

The patient usually presents within three months of delivery with severe bleeding, extensive painful bruising, bleeding from the gastrointestinal and genitourinary tract, and occasional haemarthroses. The confirmed cases presented within 3 days to 17 months of delivery. The factor VIII antibody is associated with lifethreatening haemorrhage at various sites, not necessarily affected by parturition.

Diagnosis of factor VIII antibody

The prothrombin time and thrombin time are normal but the partial thromboplastin time is very long (see Fig. 1.5, Ch. 1). The partial thromboplastin time is not corrected by the addition of normal plasma or factor VIII.

The potency of the antibody is determined by an assay in which the ability of concentrations of the patient's plasma to destroy VIIIC is observed, the result being expressed in u/ml. The unit is defined as that quantity of antibody contained in undiluted patient's plasma which will destroy 0.5 i.u. VIIIC in 4 hours at 37° (Ingram et al 1982).

Management

Any woman who develops such an antibody should be under the care of a unit expert in the management of coagulation problems. Treatment of the acute bleeding episode is difficult because conventional amounts of factor VIII may just enhance antibody formation and fail to control the bleeding. Immunosuppressive agents in combination with corticosteroids have been suggested to reduce the antibody production and there are reports of a decrease or disappearance of the antibody in response to such treatment (Coller et al 1981). In one reported case (Reece et al 1982), after failure of factor VIII concentrate and fresh plasma, improvement in the clinical status was achieved by administration of an anti-inhibitor coagulation complex (Autoplex), a preparation of pooled fresh plasma containing precursors and activated clotting factors. The mechanism of action of Autoplex is unknown. It does not suppress or destroy the inhibitor but seems to control the acute haemorrhagic diathesis (Reece et al 1982).

The natural history is for the antibody to disappear gradually usually within two years. Women should be advised to avoid further pregnancy until their coagulation is back to normal, although in the one documented case where conception occurred, the antibody disappeared during the course of the pregnancy (Voke & Letsky 1977).

REFERENCES

Atlas M, Barkai G, Menczer J, Houlu N, Lieberman P 1982 Thrombotic thrombocytopenic purpura in pregnancy. British Journal of Obstetrics and Gynaecology 89: 476–479

Ayromlooi J 1978 A new approach to the management of immunologic thrombocytopenic purpura in pregnancy. American Journal of Obstetrics and Gynecology 130: 235–236

Bell W R 1977 Hematologic abnormalities in pregnancy. Medical Clinics of North America 61: 1–165

Boey M L, Colaco C B, Gharavi A E, Elkon K B, Loizou S, Hughes G R V 1983 Thrombosis in systemic lupus erythematosus: striking association with the presence of circulating lupus anticoagulant. British Medical Journal 287: 1021–1023

Bonnar J 1981. In: Bloom A L, Thomas D P (eds) Haemostasis and coagulation disorders in pregnancy. Churchill Livingstone, Edinburgh

Boxer M, Ellman C, Carvallho A 1976 The lupus anticoagulant. Arthritis and Rheumatism 19: 1244–1248

Carloss H W, McMillar R, Crosby W H 1980 Management of pregnancy in women with immune thrombocytopenic purpura. Journal of the American Medical Association 244: 2756–2758

Carreras L O, Vermylen J, Spitz B, Van Assche A 1981 Lupus anticoagulant and inhibition of prostacyclin formation in patients with repeated abortion, intrauterine growth retardation and intrauterine death. British Journal of Obstetrics and Gynaecology 88: 890–894

Coller B S et al 1981 Normal pregnancy in a patient with a prior postpartum factor VIII inhibitor: With observations on pathogenesis and prognosis. Blood 58: 619–624

Difino S M, Lachant N A, Kirchner J J, Gottlieb A J 1980 Adult ITP — clinical findings and response to therapy. American Journal of Medicine 69: 430–432

Epstein R D, Longer E L, Conbey J T 1950 Congenital thrombocytopenic purpura. Purpuric haemorrhage in pregnancy and the newborn. American Journal of Medicine 9: 44–56

Fine L G et al 1981 Systemic lupus erythematosus in pregnancy. Annals of Internal Medicine 94: 667–677

Grigor R R, Shervington P C, Hughes G R V, Hawkins D F 1977 Outcome of pregnancy in systemic lupus erythematosus. Proceedings of the Royal Society of Medicine 70: 99–100

Hegde U M, Bowes A, Powell D K, Joyner M V 1981 Detection of platelet-bound and serum antibodies in thrombocytopenia by enzyme-linked assay. Vox Sanguinis 41: 306–312

Hegde U M, Gordon Smith E C, Worlledge S M 1977 Platelet antibodies in thrombocytopenic patients. British Journal of Haematology 35: 113–122

Hellman R M, Jackson D V, Buss D H 1980 Thrombotic thrombocytopenic purpura and hemolytic-uremic syndrome in HLA identical siblings. Annals of Internal Medicine 93: 283–284

Houser M T, Fish A J, Tagatz G E, Williams P P, Michael A F 1980 Pregnancy and systemic lupus erythematosus. American Journal of Obstetrics and Gynecology 138: 409–413

Hubbard H C, Portnoy B 1979 Systemic lupus erythematosus in pregnancy treated with plasmapheresis. British Journal of Dermatology 101: 87–89

115

Hughes G R V 1979 Systemic lupus erythematosus. In: Connective tissue diseases. Blackwell Scientific Publications, Oxford

Hughes G R V 1983 Thrombosis, abortion, cerebral disease and the lupus anticoagulant. British Medical Journal 287: 1088–1089

Imbach P, Barandum S, d'Apuzzo V 1981 High dose intravenous gammaglobulin for idiopathic thrombocytopenic purpura in childhood. Lancet i: 1128–1231

Ingram G I L, Brozovic M, Slater N G P 1982 Thrombotic thrombocytopenic purpura and the haemolytic uraemic syndrom. In: Bleeding disorders — investigation and management. Blackwell Scientific Publications, Oxford, p 131–135

Kelton J C, Blanchette V S, William E W 1980 Neonatal thrombocytopenia due to passive immunisation. Prenatal diagnosis and distinction between maternal platelet alloantibodies and autoantibodies. New England Journal of Medicine 302: 1401–1403

Kelton J G et al 1982 The prenatal prediction of thrombocytopenia in infants of mothers with clinically diagnosed immune thrombocytopenia. American Journal of Obstetrics and Gynecology 144: 449–454

Kwaan H C, Guillermo A, Potter E, Cutting H and Stanzler R 1968 The nature of vascular lesion in thrombotic thrombocytopenic purpura. Annals of Internal Medicine 68: 1169–1170

Van Leeuwen E F, Helmer Horsten F M, Engelfrat C P, Von Dem Borne A E K 1981 Maternal autoimmune thrombocytopenia and the newborn. British Medical Journal 283: 104

Lian E C-Y, Harkness D R, Byrnes J J, Wallach H, Nunez R 1979 Presence of a platelet aggregating factor in the plasma of patients with thrombotic thrombocytopenic purpura (TTP) and its inhibition by normal plasma. Blood 53: 333–338

Lubbe W F, Butler W S, Palmer S J, Liggins G C 1983b Fetal survival after prednisone suppression of maternal lupus anticoagulant. Lancet i: 1361–1363

McMillan R 1981 Chronic idiopathic thrombocytopenic purpura. New England Journal of Medicine 304: 1135–1147

Machin S J, Defrey N G, Vermylen J, Willoughby M L N 1981 Prostacyclin deficiency in thrombotic thrombocytopenic purpura (TTP) and the haemolytic uraemic syndrom (HUS). British Journal of Haematology 49: 141–142

Marchesi D, Parbtani A, Frampton G, Livio M, Remuzzi G, Cameron J S 1981 Thrombotic tendency in systemic lupus erythematosis. Lancet i: 719

Marengo Rowe A J, Murff G, Leveson J E, Cook J 1972 Haemophilia-like disease associated with pregnancy. Obstetrics and Gynecology 40: 56–64

May H V Jr, Harbert F M Jr, Thornton W N J 1976 Thrombotic thrombocytopenic purpura associated with pregnancy. American Journal of Obstetrics and Gynecology 126: 452–458

Morgenstern G R, Measday B, Hegde U M 1983 Autoimmune thrombocytopenia in pregnancy: New approach to management. British Medical Journal 287: 584

Mueh J R, Erbst K D, Rapaport S I 1980 Thrombosis in patients with lupus anticoagulant. Annals of Internal Medicine 92: 156–159

Newland A L, Treleaven J G, Minchinton R M, Waters A H 1983 High-dose intravenous IgG in adults with autoimmune thrombocytopenia. Lancet i: 84–87

Nilsson I M, Astedt B, Hedner U, Berezin D 1975 Intrauterine death and circulating anticoagulant 'antithromboplastin'. Acta medica scandinavica 197: 153–159

O'Brien J R 1954 An acquired coagulation defect in a woman. Journal of Clinical Pathology 7: 22

Perkins R P (1979) Thrombocytopenia in obstetric syndromes: a review. Obstetric and Gynecological Survey 34: 101–114

Pitkin R M 1980 Drugs in pregnancy. In: Quilligan E J, Kretchmer N (eds) Fetal and maternal medicine. Wiley Medical Publications, New York, p 385–402

Pritchard M H, Jessop J D, Trenchard P M, Whittaker J A 1978 Systemic lupus erythematosus repeated abortions and thrombocytopenia. Annals of Rheumatic Diseases 37: 476–478

Reece E A, Fox H E, Rapoport F 1982: Factor VIII inhibitor: a cause of severe postpartum haemorrhage. American Journal of Obstetrics and Gynecology 144: 985–987

Salama A, Mueller-Eckhardt C, Kiefel V 1983 Effect of intravenous immunoglobulin in immune thrombocytopenia. Lancet ii: 193–195

Scott J R, Cruickshank D P, Lochencu R M D, Pitkin R M, Warenski J C 1980 Fetal platelet counts in the obstetric management of immunologic thrombocytopenic purpura. American Journal of Obstetrics and Gynecology 136: 495–499

Stratta P, Canavese C, Bussolino P, Mansueto M G, Gagliardi G, Vercellone A 1983 Haemolytic abortive syndrome. Lancet i: 424–425

Stuart M J, Gross S J, Elrad H, Graeber J E 1982 Effects of acetyl salicylatic acid ingestion on maternal and neonatal haemostasis. New England Journal of Medicine 307: 909–912

Tancer M L 1960 Idiopathic thrombocytopenic purpura and pregnancy. Report of 5 new cases and review of the literature. American Journal of Obstetrics and Gynecology 79: 148–153

Terao T et al 1981 Pregnancy complicated by idiopathic thrombocytopenic purpura. Journal of Obstetrics and Gynaecology 2: 1–10

Territo M, Finkelstein J, Oh O 1973 Management of autoimmune thrombocytopenia in pregnancy and the neonate. Obstetrics and Gynecology 41m: 579–582

Tozman E, Vrowitz M B, Gladman D D 1980 Systemic lupus erythromatosus and pregnancy. Journal of Rheumatology 7: 624–632

Varner M W, Meehan R T, Syrop C H, Strottmann M P Goplerud C P 1982 Pregnancy in patients with systemic lupus erythematosus. American Journal of Obstetrics and Gynecology 145: 1025–1037

Voke J, Letsky E 1977 Pregnancy and antibody to factor VIII. Journal of Clinical Pathology 30: 928–932

Webster J, Rees A J, Lewis P J, Hensby C N 1980 Prostacyclin deficiency in haemolytic uraemic syndrome. British Medical Journal 281: 271

Wenske C et al 1983 Treatment of idiopathic thrombocytopenic purpura in pregnancy by high-dose intravenous immunoglobulin. Blut 46: 347–353

Zulman J I, Talal N, Hoffman G S, Epstein W V 1980 Problems associated with the management of pregnancies in patients with systemic lupus erythematosus. Journal of Rheumatology 7: 37–55

6

Inherited coagulation defects which may complicate pregnancy and their management

The haemophilias and related bleeding disorders

The haemophilias are a group of inherited disorders associated with abnormal, reduced or absent coagulation factors VIII or IX with an incidence around 1 in 10 000 in developed countries (Jones 1977). The most common is haemophilia A which is associated with deficiency of factor VIII; about one-sixth of the 3000–4000 cases in Great Britain today have a condition known as Christmas disease due to a lack of coagulation factor IX (haemophilia B). Clinical manifestations of the two conditions are indistinguishable, the symptoms and signs being variable and depending on the degree of the lack of the coagulation factors concerned. Severe disease with frequent spontaneous bleeding (particularly haemarthroses) is associated with clotting factor levels of 0–1%. Less severe disease is found in subjects with clotting factors of 1–4%. Spontaneous bleeding and severe bleeding after minor trauma are rare events in cases with coagulation factor levels between 5 and 30%; the danger is that the condition may be clinically silent but during the course of major surgery or following trauma, such subjects behave as if with the very severest forms of haemophilia. Unless the defect is recognised and the lacking coagulation factor replaced, such patients will continue to bleed. The inheritance of both haemophilias is X-linked — recessive — being expressed in the male and carried by the female.

The risks in pregnancy for a female carrier of haemophilia are twofold:

1. She may, by process of Lyonisation, have a very low factor VIII or IX level which puts her at risk of excessive bleeding, particularly following a traumatic or surgical delivery.

2. Fifty per cent of her male offspring will inherit haemophilia and 50% of her daughters will be carriers like herself.

Factor VIII deficiency also occurs in Von Willebrand's disease, but is rarely very severe. This condition is inherited as an autosomal dominant and accounts for approximately 10% of all inherited disorders of blood coagulation. However, because the commoner disorders of haemophilia and Christmas disease are X-linked, Von Willebrand's disease is the most common clinically significant inherited abnormality of coagulation in women (Levin 1982). Occasionally in the rare homozygous form there is severe depression of factor VIII and a major bleeding disorder results (Bloom 1981). It was first described in 1926 by Von Willebrand in members of several families in the Alond Islands, who had an unusual bleeding disorder characterised by epistaxes, ease of bruising, menorrhagia and postpartum haemorrhage. The condition was first known as 'pseudo haemophilia' despite the equal incidence in males and females and the fact that spontaneous deep tissue bleeding and haemarthroses were rare. On the other hand gastro-intestinal and superficial skin haemorrhages, were common, unlike haemophilia. Von Willebrand's disease is the only common inherited coagulation disorder associated with a prolonged bleeding time.

In vitro tests of platelet function reveal reduced retention in a glass bead column and impairment of ristocetin-induced platelet aggregation. The platelets are intrinsically normal but fail to adhere to the vascular subendothelium.

Molecular basis of the haemophilias and Von Willebrand's disease

Factor VIII circulates as a complex of two proteins of unequal size (Table 6.1). There is a low-molecular weight portion VIIIC which promotes coagulation linked to a large multimer known as Willebrand factor VIIIWF or VIIIRAg (VIII related antigen). The biosynthesis of factor VIIIC, coded for by the X-chromosome, is reduced or abnormal in haemophilia A. The larger VIIIWF/RAg serves as a 'carrier' for VIIIC, is under separate autosomal control and is unaffected in haemophilia. The reduced VIIIC in Von Willebrand's disease is controlled by the VIIIWF/RAg deficiency. VIIIC deficiency in Von Willebrand's disease can be corrected by infusion of VIIIRAg. In early studies a rise of VIIIC was induced in Von Willebrand's disease after infusion of haemophiliac plasma

Table 6.1 Factor VIII molecular complex

VIIIC	Procoagulant in plasma (detected in bioassay)	Molecular weight 293 000 X-chromosome
VIIICAg	Antigen detectable by human antibody to VIIIC Immunoradiometric assay (IRMA)	
VIIIWF	Willebrand factor Measured by bleeding time Ristocetin aggregation of platelets	Molecular weight (Polymers × 220 000) Autosome
VIIIRAg	Antigen detectable by heterologous antibody raised in rabbit to human factor VIII (IRMA)	

VIIIC + VIIIWF = complex
Molecular weight $> 1 \times 10^6$

which was totally deficient in VIIIC but had normal content of VIIIWF/RAg (see Mibashan & Millar 1983).

Factor VIIIC activity in plasma is measured in a bioassay technique by its ability to shorten the clotting time of severe haemophilic plasma. This requires a clean venepuncture because incipient coagulation in improperly collected blood may cause false high or low results. An immunoradiometric assay (IRMA) of the antigenic determinants of VIIIC (VIIICAg) has enabled measurement of the coagulant moiety of factor VIII complex by an alternative method. Human IgG antibodies which may arise against VIIIC are used to measure the molecular determinants of the small molecule concerned with coagulant activity — VIIICAg. There is good correlation between the measurement of VIIIC (bioassay) and VIIICAg (IRMA).

Factor VIIIWF, Von Willebrand factor, is measured as factor VIIIRAg — VIII related antigen — by rabbit antibodies raised against human factor VIII in an immunoassay system as ristocetin cofactor in a platelet aggregating system.

subunits. There is a small clot promoting molecule VIIIC/VIIICAg, which is abnormal or lacking in haemophilia A. This is linked to a larger multimeric molecule, factor VIIIWF/factor VIIIRAg, which is present in normal and haemophilic subjects, promotes platelet adhesion and aggregation and is reduced or defective in Von Willebrand's disease (Mibashan & Millar 1983 Tables 6.1 and 6.2).

Factor IX is a vitamin K-dependent clotting factor which is an

Table 6.2 Factor VIII complex in haemophilia A and Von Willebrand's disease

	VIIIC	VIIICAg	VIIIRAg	VIIIC VIIIRAg ratio
Haemophilia A	Low or absent	Low or absent	Normal or increased	Greatly reduced
Carriers of haemophilia A	Low or normal	Low or normal	Normal	Usually reduced
Von Willebrand's disease	Variably depressed	Variably depressed	Variably depressed in parallel with VIIIC and VIIICAg	Normal 1:1

Coagulation Problems During Pregnancy

essential cofactor in the intrinsic clotting mechanism (Table 1.2, Ch. 1). Factor IX coagulant clotting factor IXC is reduced in vitamin K insufficiency and in conditions associated with impaired hepatic function, as well as in the genetically determined Christmas disease. Low levels are therefore usual in the course of warfarin therapy (see Ch.2) and also in the newborn and fetus due to lack of vitamin K combined with immaturity of the liver. Although there is an immunoradiometric assay which will measure factor IX antigen using a human antibody to factor IXC, its usefulness is limited since around one-third of severely affected patients with Christmas disease have significant levels of functionally defective IXCAg. This crossreacting material (CRM) limits the use of IRMA in the prenatal diagnosis of Christmas disease (see below) and many cases can only be diagnosed using a factor IXC bioassay system.

Von Willebrand's disease and pregnancy

The literature on the management and outcome of pregnancy in patients with Von Willebrand's disease is not very extensive, but there does not seem to be any evidence that the presence of Von Willebrand's disease results in either increased maternal mortality or fetal loss, although there is an increased risk of postpartum haemorrhage (Levin 1982). Noller et al (1973), reporting 4 cases, found only 18 well described cases in the English Literature. More recently 7 further cases were described by Punnonen & colleagues (1981). The relatively low frequency of complications during pregnancy may reflect the relatively benign nature of this disorder in the majority of patients; the basic deficiency of factor VIII is usually only moderate and, as the normal tendency of factor VIII is to increase in concentration during pregnancy, by term the levels are near normal (Walker & Dormandy 1968, Noller et al 1973, Krishnamurthy & Miotti 1977, Punnonen et al 1981). In most patients a parallel increase in VIIIC and VIIIRAg will occur during the pregnancy, the highest levels being reached near term (Walker & Dormandy 1968).

A correction of the bleeding-time in patients with Von Willebrand's disease during pregnancy has been reported (Straus & Diamond 1963), but the bleeding time and platelet functional abnormalities are poor indicators of severity of disease, it is only those women with low factor VIIIC who are liable to suffer severe

122

postpartum haemorrhage. Patients with this disease should be investigated at regular intervals during pregnancy and, if factor VIII levels remain low, an infusion of cryoprecipitate or fresh frozen plasma should be given at the onset of labour and continued for 4–5 days postpartum to maintain the VIIIC level in the blood at 50% or above (Hathaway & Bonnar 1978). The administration of 3 units of fresh frozen plasma or 6 units of cryoprecipitate will probably produce the maximum response of which a patient is capable (Levin 1982). Such patients respond typically to the transfusion of plasma (or plasma components containing factor VIIIRAg) by producing new factor VIIIC in vivo. Concentrates of factor VIII should not be used except in emergency situations where an immediate increase in factor VIII is required because purified concentrates of factor VIII may lack the factor that is responsible for the production of new factor VIII in vivo. (Factor VIII concentrates also carry with them the increased risk of hepatitis and AIDS associated with multiple donations).

Trauma during delivery should be minimised, caesarean section can be undertaken if indicated, provided that the factor VIII level is normal. Replacement of this factor is advisable to cover surgery and until healing of the scar is established, unless levels have risen well into the normal range at the time labour begins (Krishnamurthy & Miotti 1977).

It is obvious from what has gone before that a pregnant woman with Von Willebrand's disease should be managed in a unit which has access to expert laboratory coagulation control and advice. The diagnosis of such a condition, will be difficult during the course of pregnancy because of the alterations in coagulation activity which regularly take place. If the question of Von Willebrand's disease first arises during pregnancy it would be wise to cover delivery with cryoprecipitate or fresh frozen plasma and arrange for definitive investigation to take place about three months postpartum.

Management of carriers of haemophilia in pregnancy

On average, female carriers of haemophilia A or B do not have clinical manifestations, but in rare individuals in whom the factor VIIIC or IX levels are unusually low (10 — 30% of normal), abnormal bleeding may occur after trauma or surgery. It is important to identify carriers prior to pregnancy not only to provide genetic counselling (see below) but so that appropriate provision can be made for those rare cases with pathologically low coagulation factor activity. Fortunately the level of the deficient factor tends to increase during the course of pregnancy, as in normal women.

If the factor VIII level remains low in carriers of haemophilia A, cryoprecipitate or fresh frozen plasma should be given to cover delivery and continued for 3–4 days postpartum, such that factor VIII levels are maintained above 50%. A clinical problem is more likely in carriers of factor IX deficiency (Christmas disease) than in factor VIII deficiency carriers (Levin 1982).

Techniques for the detection of carriers of factor IX deficiency have not yet been developed in the same way as for factor VIII deficiency. In the exceptionally rare situations where the factor IX level is very low and remains so during pregnancy the patient should be managed with fresh frozen plasma to cover delivery and for three or four days postpartum. This is preferable to factor IX concentrates which are prepared from multiple donations and contain factor II, VII and X as well as factor IX and therefore carry a much greater thrombogenic hazard (Hathaway & Bonnar 1978). Again these patients should be managed in a unit with access to expert advice, laboratory coagulation service, and immediate access to the appropriate plasma components required for replacement therapy.

Prenatal diagnosis of haemophilia

There are between 3000 and 4000 cases of haemophilia in Great Britain today and because of the high mutation rate, approximately one-third of cases have no known family history. Advice on family planning has been based on identification of the carrier state and the conventional counselling for a sex-linked disorder, i.e. contraception or fetal sexing by amniocentesis and termination of male pregnancies in those who would accept such an outcome.

The ratio of VIIIC to VIIIRAg may be reduced in haemophilia carriers and, together with family studies and discriminant functional analysis, has aided in their detection (see below).

With the development of fetal blood sampling techniques for the prenatal diagnosis of the haemoglobinopathies came the possibility of diagnosing other conditions, and in particular the haemophilias. However, this requires the examination of pure fetal plasma and any contamination with amniotic fluid may interfere with the measurement in question.

Carrier detection of haemophilia

In families with haemophilia or Christmas disease, carrier females are not all identifiable.

Obligate carriers (Mibashan & Millar 1983) are:

1. All daughters of a haemophiliac father.

2. A woman with more than one haemophiliac son.

3. A woman with one haemophiliac son and a proven haemophiliac relative in her own family or her mother's.

4. The relative of a haemophiliac sufferer, the male fetus of whom is found to be haemophiliac on prenatal testing.

Putative carriers are daughters of a known haemophiliac carrier who have a 50:50 chance of inheriting the abnormal X-chromosome as do their brothers. The homozygous male is easily identified, but the heterozygous female may have to be content with a statistical estimate of her genotype by discriminant analysis utilising family data and haematological investigations (see below). A further aid to carrier detection in a few females is the demonstration of a linkage between haemophilia A and a G6-PD variant, another X-linked genetic marker. Although it has proved possible to diagnose carrier status during pregnancy (Mibashan & Millar 1983) the need to make early plans for fetal sexing and to take the required blood samples required means that the status should be established before pregnancy whenever practicable.

Carrier detection is desirable because, while fetal blood sampling can detect the affected males, it is a hazardous procedure and should only be offered to reliably diagnosed carriers. In accordance with Lyon's hypothesis, the mean level of coagulation activity in a bioassay of factor VIIIC in obligate carriers is about 50% of that observed in normal females. Unfortunately, because of the wide normal range of VIIIC levels (50–200 u/dl) only a relatively small proportion of VIIIC plasma levels in obligate carriers fall below 50% of the lower range and it is of little value in identifying the majority of women at risk of transmitting haemophilia. The introduction of the measurement of a molecule biochemically related to VIIIC but having no coagulation activity — factor VIII related antigen or VIIIRAg — which is present at normal or slightly increased levels in haemophilia and haemophilia carriers, greatly improved the detection rate. The concentration of VIII procoagulant activity relative to that of factor VIIIRAg is measured. This ratio is reduced in carriers of haemophilia and a value of below 0.7 is observed in up to 85% of obligatory carriers (see Table 6.2).

The recent introduction of immunological measurement by immunoradiometric assay (IRMA) of the antigens related to VIIIC and called VIIIC antigen or VIIICAg (Peake & Bloom 1978, Lazarchick & Hoyer 1978) show that VIIIC and VIIICAg agree well in plasma but that VIIICAg, is considerably more stable and also present in serum.

The mean ratios of VIIIC to VIIIRAg and the ratio of VIIICAg to VIIIRAg are both very significantly reduced in haemophilia carriers. However, the C antigen assay is significantly less variable and more precise than the coagulation assay and since the overlap between laboratory data on normals and carriers is partly due to variance of the coagulation bioassay, the VIIICAg assay (IRMA) should be of considerable advantage. In addition it may reduce the number of duplicate assays necessary and by virtue of the stability of both VIIICAg and VIIIRAg allow samples to be sent by post to a specialist assay centre.

The prediction of the carrier state can be further improved by discriminant analysis and this has emphasised the value of VIIIC antigen assay. Factor VIIIRAg — VIIIC and VIIICAg were determined in a group of obligatory carriers and in an age-matched group of normal women (Peake et al 1981). The values were mathematically adjusted to give normal distributions and from these the statistician calculated a discriminant which separates carrier and normal groups most effectively.

The ratio of VIIICAg:VIIIRAg proved to be more discriminant than that obtained from VIIIC:VIIIRAg. For example, at a laboratory ratio of 0.6 the odds of the consultant being a carrier are 20:1 when the VIIIC antigen assay is used, but only 3:1 when the VIII clotting assay is used. The family tree is then taken into account and the laboratory date from the putative carrier determined. The laboratory and pedigree likelihood ratios are then multiplied together to calculate the final probability of carrier status (Graham et al 1980).

This has not solved the problem for many carriers because they may wish to have a son and object to the 50% chance of losing a normal male fetus. Prenatal diagnosis, until very recently, has not been thought possible because it would depend on the factor VIIIC estimation in fetal plasma. For this an absolutely pure sample of fetal blood is required because factor VIIIC is labile, destroyed when blood clots, is interfered with by amniotic fluid which has thromboplastic activity, and would be affected by admixture of maternal plasma.

The discovery in 1978 by Peake & Bloom in Cardiff, and almost simultaneously in the United States (Lazarchick & Hoyer 1978) of an VIIIC antigen VIIICAg, detectable by immunoradiometric assay (IRMA) using an antibody raised in a treated haemophiliac, appears to remove some of the problems. VIIICAg, as opposed to VIIIRAg, is reduced in haemophilic plasma to the same extent or more than VIIIC. Unlike VIIIC, it is stable, present in serum and absent from and not affected by amniotic fluid. However, this method is not applicable to all patients because difficulties may arise where an affected member of the carrrier's family has crossreacting material in their plasma which can interfere with the assay of plasma VIIICAg; fortunately in severe haemophilia this if uncommon.

In 1979 Firchein & colleagues in Connecticut published the results of the prenatal diagnosis of six cases for haemophilia using the estimation of factor VIIICAg. Three cases had low values of factor VIIICAg and normal levels of factor VIIIRAg and the pregnancies were terminated, the diagnoses being confirmed on the abortuses. The other three patients had normal values and went to term, delivering unaffected infants. These results depended on factor VIIICAg levels corrected for considerable and variable dilution of the fetal blood samples by amniotic fluid. At King's College Hospital a technique of in utero blood sampling has been developed whereby a needle, under direct vision, is placed into an umbilical vessel just above the attachment of the cord to the chorionic plate of the placenta (Rodeck & Campbell 1978). The advantage of this is that absolutely pure fetal blood, with no admixture of maternal blood or amniotic fluid, is usually obtained. There appears to be less bleeding following this method than after sampling blood from a fetal vessel on the surface of the placenta. The results of investigations of fetuses at risk for haemophilia A, in which pure fetal blood was obtained using this technique has been published (Mibashan et al 1980). Thirty-eight of 39 samples obtained at 18–20 weeks gestation were pure fetal blood uncontaminated by amniotic fluid. Factor VIIIC was estimated by a modified one-stage bioassay and factor VIIICAg measured on the same samples. There were no postoperative complications, spontaneous abortions or preterm labours. Eleven of the 39 fetuses at risk proved to be haemophiliac and the pregnancies were terminated, diagnosis being confirmed on the abortuses. The proportion is less than one would expect if all of the mothers seeking investigation were obligate carriers, but some of the mothers were only putative carriers. Five of the 12 fetuses of obligate carriers had haemophilia. The normal diagnosis has been confirmed in all those babies who have been born.

The most recent report (Mibashan & Millar 1983) gives the results of prenatal tests in 130 male fetuses at risk of haemophilia A. The analysis of the 44 cases affected — considerably less than the 50% expected if all carriers were obligate, highlights the reprieve rate among male fetuses of women who are unwilling to bring a viable haemophilic child into the world and also the inability to identify all carriers among the female population with certainty even utilising improved methods.

Prenatal diagnosis of Christmas disease — haemophilia B, factor IX deficiency — has lagged behind that of haemophilia A, partly because it is less prevalent and also because the blood sampling and assay requirements are even more stringent in view of the normally low fetal levels of factor IX. A sensitive immunoradiometric assay for factor IX Ag has been reported (Holmberg et al 1980) capable of distinguishing the normally low levels in the fetus from those with Christmas disease. Unfortunately, this is not applicable to those families who have positive crossreacting material, the incidence of which is much higher in Christmas disease than in haemophilia A (see above).

Coagulant assays of factor IX are not suitable for samples which are contaminated with amniotic fluid, but 15 cases at risk for factor IX have now been correctly diagnosed on pure fetal blood (Mibashan & Millar 1983).

Prenatal diagnosis of Von Willebrand's disease

The very severe homozygous form of this autosomal disorder is rare. In the autosomal dominant heterozygous form factor VIIIC levels are not usually low enough or clinical manifestation severe enough to prompt a family to request prenatal diagnosis. Three severe cases have been successfully diagnosed prenatally (Mibashan & Millar 1983) by testing pure fetal blood obtained at fetoscopy.

Other genetically determined haemostatic defects which can be diagnosed prenatally

Laboratory techniques can now be applied to pure fetal blood samples for the diagnosis of the rare autosomal coagulation defects and some of the serious syndromes involving platelet depletion or disordered function.

Factor XI deficiency (PTA deficiency)

This is a rare coagulation disorder less common than the haemophilias but more common than the very rare inherited deficiencies of the remaining coagulation factors. It is inherited as an autosomal recessive, usually in Jewish people and both men and women may be affected. Usually only the homozygotes have clinical evidence of a coagulation disorder though occasionally carriers may have a mild bleeding tendency. It is a mild condition in which spontaneous haemorrhages and haemarthroses are rare but the danger lies in the fact that profuse bleeding may follow major trauma or surgery if no prophylactic plasma is given. Indeed it is often diagnosed late in life following surgery in an individual who was unaware of a serious haemostatic defect. The diagnosis is made by finding a prolonged partial thromboplastin time (see Fig.1.5) with a low factor XI level in a coagulation assay system but in which all other coagulation tests are normal. Management consists of replacement with fresh frozen plasma to treat bleeding and for prophylaxis before and after surgery. In a known case of PTA deficiency it would be wise to cover delivery with plasma, whether this be by surgery or vaginal.

Fortunately the condition rarely causes problems either during pregnancy and labour or in the child; in particular prolonged bleeding at ritual circumcision is not usual. There is therefore, no justification in screening routinely for this condition either in the mother, fetus or neonate. Very occasionally, however, both in this condition and in the even more rare autosomal recessively inherited defects of coagulation factors VII, V, X, XIII, fibrinogen and factor II, families may wish to have the defect diagnosed prenatally and affected pregnancies terminated. If pure fetal blood sampling can be undertaken, all of these conditions are susceptible to prenatal diagnosis.

Platelet abnormalities

Functional defects

Serious bleeding disorders due to inherited abnormalites of platelet function are rare, the inheritance being as an autosomal recessive. Clinically the signs and symptoms are similar to those of Von Willebrand's disease with skin and mucosal haemorrhages. Spontaneous bruises are common but haemarthroses are not. Although these disorders can lead to life-threatening haemorrhage, particularly after surgery or trauma, the bleeding tendency is usually mild. The essential defect is intrinsic to the platelet. Bleeding time is prolonged and platelet function tests are abnormal, showing reduced aggregation and/or adhesion. In thrombasthenia (Glanzmann's disease), the platelets appear morphologically normal but they fail to aggregate with collagen ADP or ristocetin. In the very rare Bernard Soulier syndrome the aggregation defect is similar but the platelets have a characteristically abnormal giant appearance. Serious bleeding episodes are treated with fresh platelet concentrate infusions. Families who have one or other of these rare defects may seek termination of pregnancy because of the severity of symptoms or the difficulties arising from management. It is theoretically possible to diagnose the condition prenatally from a pure fetal blood sample, since specific membrane glycoprotein defects have been identified in both syndromes. A sensitive monoclonal immunoassay applicable to small volumes of whole fetal blood, without the necessity of separating the platelets, greatly facilitates the prenatal diagnoses in these conditions (see Mibashan & Millar 1983).

Thrombocytopenia

Genetically determined thrombocytopenia may be associated with aplastic anaemia or isolated megakaryocytic aplasia. The syndrome of absent radii with thrombocytopenia is known as the TAR syndrome: these are thought to be autosomal recessive defects and have been successfully diagnosed prenatally by examination of fetal blood samples (Alter et al 1978).

Another X-linked symptom complex is the Wiskott Aldrich syndrome comprising severe immune deficiency with thrombocytopenia. It presents in the neonatal period but is probably expressed in utero and therefore susceptible to diagnosis prenatally.

pregnancies at risk reported so far have been female and were not examined further (Mibashan and Millar 1983). Fanconi's anaemia, a familial autosomal recessively inherited condition, is a syndrome of aplastic anaemia with varying skeletal and other physical anomalies. Although thrombocytopenia is the earliest and dominant feature of marrow aplasia, presentation is usually delayed until at least three or four years of age, so that intrauterine diagnosis by detecting thrombocytopenia in fetal blood is precluded. However, the diagnosis has been made on the basis of excessive chromosomal breaks in chemically treated amniotic fluid fibroblast cultures (Auerbach et al 1981). A more rapid result could be obtained by using fetoscopic blood for culture of fetal cells (Mibashan & Millar 1983).

The future

Recently there has been an explosion of progress in the knowledge of human molecular genetics. There has been a change of emphasis in the analysis of human genetic disease from the clinical, cellular and biochemical levels to the molecular level. During the last few years it has become possible to analyse the fine structure of human genes using recombinant DNA and molecular hybridisation techniques. The molecular basis for at least some genetic disorders has been established. For a review of the techniques involved and their application to clinical practice the reader is referred to Weatherall (1982). The possibility of identifying haemophilia carriers, as well as affected fetuses, by direct analysis of DNA is an increasingly real one. Molecular cloning of the gene for factor IX has already been undertaken (Choo et al 1982) and in Christmas disease specific changes in the gene for factor IX have been identified in a special subgroup of patients (Gianelli et al 1983). It is thought that similar success in the investigation of the gene for factor VIII will soon be achieved (Bloom 1983).

Fetal sexing may be determined at a much earlier stage of pregnancy than is possible by analysis of amniotic fluid fibroblasts by DNA analysis of chorionic biopsy material obtained at 8–10 weeks gestation (Rodeck & Morsmen 1983, Old et al 1982).

It would appear from these collected results that obstetric and haematalogical skills should be integrated and developed, and particularly that more obstetricians should learn how to obtain pure fetal tissue samples.

Coagulation Problems During Pregnancy

REFERENCES

Alter B P, Potter N U, Li F P 1978 Classification and aetiology of the aplastic anaemias. Clinics in Haematology 7: 431–465

Auerbach A D, Adler B, Chaganti R S K 1981 Prenatal and postnatal diagnosis and carrier detection of Fanconi anaemia by a cytogenetic method. Pediatrics 67: 128–135

Bloom A L 1981 Inherited disorders of blood coagulation. In: Bloom A L, Thomas D P (eds) Haemostasis and thrombosis. Churchill Livingstone, Edinburgh, p 321–370

Bloom A L 1983 Benefits of cloning genes for clotting factors, Nature 303: 474–475

Choo K H, Gould K G, Rees D J G, Brownlee G G 1982 Molecular cloning of the gene for human antihaemophilic factor IX. Nature 299: 178–180

Daker M 1983 Chorionic tissue biopsy in the first trimester of pregnancy. British Journal of Obstetrics and Gynaecology 90: 193–195

Firshein S I et al 1979 Prenatal diagnosis of classic haemophilia. New England Journal of Medicine 300: 937–941

Giannelli F, Choo K H, Rees D J G, Boyd Y, Rizza C R, Brownlee G G 1983 Gene deletions in patients with haemophilia B and antifactor IX antibodies. Nature 303: 181–182

Graham J B, Barrow E S, Flyer P, Dawson D V, Elston R C 1980 Identifying carriers of mild haemophilia. British Journal of Haematology 44: 671–678

Hathaway W E, Bonnar J 1978 Hereditary bleeding defects. In: Perinatal coagulation, Grune and Stratton, New York, p 106–107

Holmberg L et al 1980 Prenatal diagnosis of haemophilia B, by an immunoradiometric assay of factor IX. Blood 56: 397–401

Jones P 1977 Developments and problems in the management of haemophilia. Seminars in Haematology 14: 375–390

Joyer L W et al 1979 Prenatal evaluation of fetus at risk for severe Von Willebrand's disease. Lancet ii: 191–192

Krishnamurthy M, Miotti A B 1977 Von Willebrand's disease and pregnancy. Obstetrics and Gynaecology 49: 244–247

Lazarchick J, Hoyer L W 1978 Immunoradiometric measurement of the factor VIII procoagulant antigen. Journal of Clinical Investigation 62: 1048–1052

Levin J 1982 Disorders of blood coagulation and platelets. In: Burrow G N, Ferris T F (eds) Medical complications during pregnancy, 2nd edn. W B Saunders & Co, p 70–73

Mibashan R S, Millar D S 1983 Fetal haemophilia and allied bleeding disorders. British Medical Bulletin 39. No. 4 392–398

Mibashan R S, et al 1980 Dual diagnosis of prenatal haemophilia A by measurement of fetal factor VIIIC and VIIIC antigen (VIIICAg). Lancet ii: 994–997

Noller K L, Bowie E J W, Kempers R D, Owen C A 1973 Von Willebrand's disease in pregnancy. Obstetrics and Gynaecology 41: 865–872

Old J M, Ward R H T, Petrou M, Karagözlu F, Modell B M, Weatherall D J 1982 First trimester fetal diagnosis for haemoglobinopathies: three cases. Lancet ii: 1413–1416

Peake I R, Bloom A L 1978 Immunoradiometric measurement of procoagulant factor VIII antigen in plasma and serum and its reduction in haemophilia. Lancet i: 473–475

Peake I R, Newcombe R G, Davies B L, Furlong R A, Ludlam C A, Bloom A L 1981 Carrier detection in haemophilia A by immunological measurement of factor VIII related antigen (VIIIRAg) and factor VIII clotting antigen VIIICAg. British Journal of Haematology 48: 651–660

Punnonen R, Nyman D, Grönroos M, Wallen O 1981 Von Willebrand's disease and pregnancy. Acta obstetrica gynecologica scandinavica 60: 507–509

Rodeck C H, Morsmen J 1983 First trimester chorion biopsy. British Medical Bulletin 39: No.4, 338–342

Rodeck C H, Campbell S 1978 Sampling pure fetal blood by fetoscopy in second trimester of pregnancy. British Medical Journal ii: 728–730

Rodeck C G, Nicolaides K 1983 Fetoscopy and fetal tissue sampling. British Medical Bulletin 39: No.4 332–337

Straus H S, Diamond L K 1963 Elevation of factor VIII (antihaemophilic factor) during pregnancy in normal persons and in a patient with Von Willebrand's disease. New England Journal of Medicine 269: 1251–1252

Walker E H, Dormandy K Y 1968 The management of pregnancy in Von Willebrand's disease. Journal of Obstetrics and Gynaecology of the British Commonwealth 75: 459–463

Weatherall D J 1982 The new genetics and clinical practice. Nuffield Provincial Hospitals Trust

Index

Index

23